The Truth about Tummy Time

THE TRUTH ABOUT TUMMY TIME

A PARENT'S GUIDE TO SIDS, THE BACK TO SLEEP PROGRAM, CAR SEATS AND MORE.

Stephanie J. Pruitt, PT, CKTP

authorHOUSE®

AuthorHouse™
1663 Liberty Drive
Bloomington, IN 47403
www.authorhouse.com
Phone: 1-800-839-8640

First published by AuthorHouse   07/01/2011

ISBN: 978-1-4634-0874-9 (sc)
ISBN: 978-1-4634-0872-5 (ebk)

Library of Congress Control Number: 2011908281

Printed in the United States of America

Contents

Preface

Before my first child was born, I, like many new mothers, prepared for the arrival of my baby by reading every book available and listening to endless advice from those around me. One thing I remember hearing was "Never wake a sleeping baby." After he was born, I heeded this advice and was very particular about not messing with my son while he was asleep—outside of checking on him frequently to make sure he was okay. At our four-month check up, the doctor told me that the back of my son's head was flat and that I needed to go see a physical therapist.

First of all, I was offended! My baby was perfect; there was nothing wrong with his head. Second of all, I *am* a physical therapist and certainly didn't need to go see one! Granted, at that time, I worked with adults. Once I left his office, I took a good look at my son's head and realized he was right. It was flat on one side. It wasn't until then that it occurred to me that my baby always lay on the same side of his head when he slept. In every picture we took of him, his head was turned that way. I was so concerned about waking my baby, that I left him alone while he slept even though his position didn't change. In addition, I let him spend a lot of time in a soft bouncer and car seat. If he fell asleep in the car seat, I would simply put the car seat in the crib until he woke up. He spent a lot of time sleeping and playing in the bouncer as well as eating all of his meals there. The bouncer and his car seat reinforced that same favorite position.

No one advised me to rotate my baby from side to side to ensure his head would form correctly. The nurses at the hospital

1

did not instruct me in proper sleeping positions, nor did anyone mention anything about the Back-to-Sleep program. The only reason I put my son on his back to sleep was because of the vague references I'd heard to "always put your baby on his back to sleep" and the little "back to sleep" logo on his diapers. Not one person or one source of information I read covered this topic in proper detail. I had to consider it was possible I didn't read *everything* there was to read, and equally possible, I was too tired to read anything at all once the baby arrived. I guess everyone assumed I knew. And I clearly didn't realize how important the position my baby spent most of his time in was.

I started rotating my son to different positions—away from his favorite side. During my routine checks on him while he slept, I would rotate his head off the flat spot, as he always found his way back there. At that point, I was more concerned with rounding his head out than waking him up. Interestingly enough, he didn't wake up when I messed with him. Slowly, his head rounded out, and the flat spot got smaller. He is now ten years old, and unless you know where to look, you wouldn't notice that he ever had a problem. What is more, his development took off once I started putting him in different positions. He started rolling and developing strength in his back and neck muscles from lying on his stomach. These important tools of development did not occur before I started changing his position. He met all the other milestones on time and is now a great athlete with well-balanced strength and coordination. In school, he is doing very well in all his subjects, displaying no indication of cognitive deficits. My interest in pediatrics grew after his birth, so I decided to switch my specialty to Pediatric Physical Therapy.

When my second baby was born, he was five weeks' premature and spent eight days in the neonatal intensive care unit (NICU). The nurses there would routinely rotate my son to each side, his stomach, and his back. I was concerned about placing him on his stomach because of his prematurity, but when I asked our nurse about this position, she said the nurses found babies don't struggle as much to breathe when they are lying on their stomachs. "When they are really struggling or upset, we put them on their stomachs, and they consistently calm down and breathe easier."

I emulated this pattern at home with this logic: *If the NICU nurses, who worked with babies every day, recommended it, then it was good enough for me.* Considering the babies they were working with were at high risk for complications, I thought, who better would know how to care for an infant? Consequently, my second son has a perfectly rounded head. He was a little behind meeting his milestones, because of his prematurity, not because of any lack of opportunity to develop muscle balance; I made sure I changed his position every time I put him down.

Interestingly, my second son had a very unusual crawling pattern. He would sit on his right hip and propel himself with the left foot and right arm. As a pediatric physical therapist, I knew how important crawling was for development, so I would follow him around the house trying to correct it, but as you can imagine, that was exhausting. So, I waited until he was a little older and could understand my instruction and then encouraged him to crawl "like a puppy" on all fours. We played this game for several months, practicing this normal crawling pattern, to ensure that his brain received the essential connections that crawling creates between the left and right brain. Today, at eight years old, he is also a natural athlete and an excellent student.

When I gave birth to my third son, there was no doubt in my mind how to ensure the best outcome again. He was also five weeks premature and had the same unusual crawling pattern. (I joke that my second son left hieroglyphics on the inside to give my third son instructions.) We went through the same drill of the crawling game once he was old enough to understand the instructions. He is now six years old and lights up the soccer field with grace and agility. He is starting kindergarten this year, and I expect he will also follow in his brothers' footsteps in being a good student.

I always tell people that my children are the biggest source of education in my practice. In addition to their similarities, each of them developed in very different ways, so they have been a wealth of information. Watching them intrigued me and motivated me to dig for more information. Once I knew what to do to promote their development, it was actually easy!

As a mother and a pediatric physical therapist, I have noticed a trend in the last nine years—and as an instructor of other physical therapists, I hear from my colleagues from around the country that they are seeing the same trend: Almost universally, parents are concerned about sudden infant death syndrome (SIDS). And for children, today's daily routine involves hours upon hours in car seats, soft bouncers, plush swings, and cushy mattresses. As a result, I am seeing an influx of patients who have misshapen heads and shortened neck muscles; who are developmentally delayed; and who later have sensory integration issues, fine motor delays, and difficulty in school with reading and handwriting. When parents bring their infants into the clinic for a physical therapy evaluation, they all ask me the same question: Is it safe to put my baby on her stomach to sleep—what about SIDS? Most parents tell me that their babies spend little to no time on their stomachs and never have since birth.

Because of these two trends—the developmental issues I'm seeing as a PT, and the fact that parents today are almost universally taught to avoid putting their infants on their stomachs, I became motivated to look for a pattern. I embarked on a project that involved intensive research of the issues of placement, developmental delay, and SIDS. The end product of that research is this book, a concise, easy-to-follow guide that addresses all the questions I hear repeatedly in the clinic.

I had these questions, myself, as a new mother, and I would have loved an easy-to-understand, easy-to-read resource to answer them. It is my hope that this book will greatly reduce not only the uncertainty and fears around caring for infants, but also the rate of the growing epidemic of certain infant disorders that are entirely preventable through a little education and know-how.

Introduction

If you were to ask your mother or grandmother, "What position did you put your babies in when you put them down to sleep?" You might get an answer that would surprise you. I asked my mother a few years ago what position she put my sisters and me to sleep in and she replied, "The doctors told us to put babies on their side to sleep, so if you threw up, you wouldn't choke." I also asked my grandmother what position she put her babies in and she said, "We were always told to rotate our babies from side to side until they were strong enough to move around on their own. Then we let them sleep in whatever position they got themselves into." She explained further that rotating the baby in this fashion ensured the head would stay round.

Today, if you ask new mothers what positions their babies slept in, almost all of them would probably say they placed their babies on their backs to sleep. This change in thinking occurred with the introduction of the National Institute of Child Health and Human Development's Back to Sleep program in 1994, in an effort to reduce the number children who died from sudden infant death syndrome (SIDS). Preliminary data collected under the leadership of the National Institute of Child Health and Human Development indicated that the program was successful with a reduction in the rate of sudden infant death, but it is questionable if the Back to Sleep program can take full credit for this reduction. In the last two decades, there have been advancements in technology, advocacy for screening, as well as a massive research effort contributing to the knowledgebase in caring for infants. Many previously unknown factors are now easily detected and treated that could have resulted in death in earlier years.

For all the wonderful things this era of medical advancement has brought in the arena of infant care, the fear of SIDS is still in the forefront of many new parents' minds. This apprehension directly influences how parents care for their babies today. In addition, the introduction of contemporary safety standards for infant transportation coupled with modern conveniences, babies are spending more and more time confined on their backs in car seats, swings, bouncers, and various other apparatuses. This combination of uncertainty and confinement is creating a dramatic rise in certain infant diagnoses such as developmental delay, torticollis, and plagiocephaly. It is difficult to radically change one aspect of infant care without influencing other areas. We are currently seeing this effect.

The first purpose of *The Truth About Tummy Time* is to provide an overview of how your baby should be developing with a discussion of physiology and development The second is to explore the leading theories on sudden infant death syndrome and the Back to Sleep program. The third is to discuss other factors that are contributing to the reduction in the SIDS rate besides back-sleeping. You will also find information on available screening tests in the event you would like to obtain further information about your own baby's health. The final purpose is to increase awareness of the infant diagnoses that are on the rise. These problems are thought to be more prevalent today as a direct result of the Back to Sleep program and the increased use of car seats, bouncers, swings, and the like.

It is my hope to answer your questions about these areas while giving helpful suggestions from a pediatric physical therapist's standpoint on the physical development and safety of your child. Ultimately, my goal is to reduce the rising trends we're seeing in pediatric physical therapy in conjunction with ongoing efforts to lower the rate of SIDS. The conflict between these two valuable fronts requires resolution so that attention to one does not cause an increase in the other.

ABOUT THE TEXT

As you read, you will notice I have varied the use *he/him* and *she/her* in referring to babies and parents, in an attempt be inclusive of each gender. These are generic references and not indicative of a certain topic in relation to a specific gender.

1

Physiology and Development

The most important thing to remember about development is that it is defined in a range. Every baby develops at his or her own rate. There are several factors that affect this range. For instance, if your baby is born prematurely, her age is adjusted for how early she was. My son was born five weeks early; so at five weeks old, he was behaving, for the most part, like a newborn baby. If a baby is born at thirty weeks' gestation, the development will be delayed ten weeks, so you could expect your baby to be about two and a half months behind in meeting developmental milestones. This is all based on a forty-week gestation or pregnancy. It is not to say that a full-term baby (thirty-eight to forty weeks' gestation) will hit the mark every time either. If you talked with a group of mothers, some would say that their babies did things earlier, others later than your baby. That is perfectly normal. It is important to note that growth and development indicate health inside the body. Typically, most healthy children reach the same level of development by three years old.

Human development refers to the natural changes that occur in a person's life from conception to death. These changes can be *progressive*, *reorganizational*, or *regressive* across the lifespan. *Progressive* changes occur during growth from infancy to adulthood. It is the maturation process of the body. *Reorganization* can occur in the event of an injury with the body repairing and/or adapting to a weakness or loss of function of the body's tissue. Another example of reorganization is being pregnant. Your body adapts to the growing weight of the baby by shifting your center of gravity so you can balance. The muscles and bones of the body must adapt to this new position until the baby is born, then revert back to the original pre-pregnancy state. *Regressive* changes occur as we age and our bodies begin the normal breakdown process. Think of development as a change in form and function.[1] At different times in your life, your body is required to do different things; therefore, it must adapt at various ages to accommodate these movement patterns, the way your body moves in a coordinated way to accomplish a task.

There are several factors that affect human development. Genetics, of course, has a lot to do with the way you develop. Your genes direct how fast you mature, as well as what traits you will take on as a child and later as an adult.

Nutrition plays a key role as well. Food supplies the body with nutrients and energy to move, to repair tissues in the body, and is one of the factors instrumental in establishing the body's chemistry. With balanced internal chemistry, the body will progress properly through growth spurts and maintain its capability in functional activities like movement.

The environment plays a very big role. Babies are raised differently in different cultures, which affects when they do the things they do. One example is crowded orphanages. If babies are not given the opportunity to get out of their cribs and explore, they will not develop normally. It would be very difficult to develop crawling skills, walking skills, or basic strength if you were not given the occasion to get out of bed.

Lastly, infection, trauma at birth or birth defects, and injury will also affect the rate of development, especially if lengthy hospital stays are involved. Most of the time, babies are confined in these instances in order to keep tubes in place and lines where they are suppose to be. These conditions can cause development to be delayed or impaired.[1]

PROCESS OF DEVELOPMENT

Let's discuss the developmental sequence a little. It is important to note that movement occurs in a specific order. In a basic building-block process, every skill builds on what happened before it. We talk a lot about *motor milestones,* because that is how the medical community evaluates how a baby is progressing.

Development starts at the head and progresses down to the feet. The term for this progression is *cephalocaudal.* It means the first thing a baby develops is head control. Next, development progresses from *proximal* to *distal*—or control of the trunk (proximal) outward to purposefully using the hands and feet (distal). So, first the baby learns to control her head, and then to control her trunk, then shoulders and pelvis, and finally arms, legs, hands, and feet.

Babies are born asymmetrical, meaning the head is turned to one side, and become more symmetrical by four months. This has to do with strength and control of opposing muscles as well as reflexes and gravity. As a baby gets older, she deals with things in midline and uses both sides of the body together—symmetrically. You will see this as she brings toys to the center of her body to observe and play with them using both hands.

In addition, babies develop gross motor skills first and then fine motor skills. This means that they use their large muscle groups first—to do big movements like rolling and sitting up—before the small muscle groups like the ones in the hands for grasping objects and coloring.

Then there is a *kinesiologic* or movement sequence. The fetal position is synonymous with the baby's totally flexed position as a newborn. Everything is all curled up like a little ball. As gravity starts to pull on the baby, she stretches out and moves into an extended position. Strength is built by moving the body against gravity from different positions—lying on the stomach, lying on the back, etc. A baby begins to build that strength by actively extending the head and rotating it from side to side while lying on her stomach. As strength increases in the neck muscles, head control is established. Without head control, the child cannot get necessary stimulation from her sense of balance, resulting in low muscle tone and muscle weakness. The ability to lift one's head is decisive to muscle tone, posture, and further development.[2]

In harmony with developmental sequence, the baby's extension against gravity moves down the body. An infant first develops head control, then trunk control, and so on by lying on the stomach. Once extensor strength is established, the baby begins to develop flexor strength. There must be muscle balance between the flexor and extensor muscles for a baby to develop well-rounded strength. Flexors bend a joint and extensors straighten a joint. These movements of bending and straightening are essential for the baby to move to the next level of skill acquisition.[1]

Think about this. If a baby is always on her back, how can she develop muscle strength of the head, neck, and back muscles against gravity? If she is never placed on her stomach, how can she develop the necessary strength to lift her head up off the floor? And if this process of building strength is thwarted, do you think she will meet her motor milestones on time?

Finally, babies move from mobility to stability. They first learn to move, and then they learn to stabilize. Mobility is movement. Stability is the ability to hold a posture. This process is called *postural control*. Stability and mobility develop incrementally, as they must occur together for a well-coordinated outcome. Once the body can hold a posture, more-purposeful movement can occur. For example, a baby must first learn to balance while sitting, before she can move her arms and legs around to reach a toy or turn in a circle to see her mom.[1]

This sequence has to occur in this order for milestones to be met. If any component of this process is hampered, not allowed, stifled, or skipped, you could see delays or problems occur. Understand that you can't rush development. It has to occur at the baby's own pace in this sequential way—no matter what age the baby is. If your child cannot hold her head up, it is not realistic to expect her to be able to roll by herself. If your child is not able to sit up on her own, it is not realistic to expect her to be able to walk. You have all heard the old adage you must first walk before you can run. It is absolutely true!

Below is an outline of the range-of-motor milestones that allied health professionals use when determining if a baby is developing on target. [3]

0 Months
- Lifts and rotates head while lying on the stomach
- Holds back in rounded position in supported sitting
- Bends and straightens legs while on back
- Rolls onto back from side-lying position
- Bends and straightens arms while on back
- Displays grasp reflex
- Holds rattle briefly

1 Month
- Child holds head at 45-degree angle in supported sitting position
- Watches a rattle by turning head from side to side through full range
- Lacks sufficient strength to hold head up when pulled into sitting position

2 Months
- Takes steps when held and leaned forward in standing position (walking reflex)
- Holds head in midline while pulling up to sit
- Raises head at midline and holds briefly when suspended vertically
- Looks at hands
- Briefly bears weight with knees flexed and feet flat when held standing
- Grasps rattle when hand is brushed with it and holds for 30 seconds.

3 Months

- Baby holds head upright when body is tilted from side to side
- Extends back briefly in supported sitting position
- Child brings both hands together to midline to reach for a toy, with head in midline
- Reaches for and shakes rattle

4 Months

- Child rotates head toward toy when in supported sitting position
- Props on arms and elevates head and trunk while on stomach
- Rolls to side, reaching with opposite arm
- Extends arms and legs off surface, briefly, while on stomach

5 Months

- Maintains balance in sitting position for brief periods
- Brings feet to mouth or grabs feet with hands
- Raises arms and legs in smooth, fluid motion toward toy
- Grasps string and pulls toy toward self on stomach
- Grasps cube in hand and holds for a short period

6 Months

- Reflexively protects self with arm when losing balance to the side while sitting
- Reaches for toys while balanced in sitting position
- Assists with head and arms when pulled up into sitting position
- Sits unsupported for a moment
- Raises trunk from surface, shifts weight, and reaches for toy on stomach
- Grasps both feet with hands and holds them while on back
- Pushes up on arms while on stomach—push-ups
- Holds and moves rattle purposefully

7 Months
- Leans over to retrieve toy and returns to upright sitting while maintaining balance
- Rolls from back to stomach on both sides
- Grasps cube with thumb, first and second fingers
- Transfers one cube to other hand and picks up a second cube

8 Months
- Uses arms to move forward 3 feet on stomach
- Grasps food with raking motion of fingers
- Crumples paper using palms—one or both hands
- Pokes finger in hole of pegboard
- Removes pegs from pegboard

9 Months
- Keeps head upright when leaning forward while sitting
- Maintains balance sitting while playing with toy
- Raises and bears weight on hands and knees, briefly, while rocking back and forth
- Creeps forward 5 feet on hands and knees
- Scoots on bottom 3 feet
- Turns body around by pivoting in sitting
- Raises to a standing position using stable object for support
- Holds cube in each hand and brings to midline
- Claps hands 3 times

10 Months
- Reflexively reaches backward to protect self from falling in sitting
- Raises up to a sitting position from stomach to reach toy
- Creeps over obstacle to get toy
- Takes 4 steps sideways while holding on to table
- Stoops and recovers while holding table
- Releases cube into your hand when asked

11 Months
- Pivots 180 degrees in sitting position
- Stands alone briefly by freeing hand and body from table
- Child takes 4 alternating steps in place or forward when held standing

12 Months
- Catches a rolled ball in sitting position without losing balance
- Opens board book
- Stirs spoon in a cup
- Turns bottle, dumps out food

This is the development you can expect if your baby is given the opportunity to move and develop muscle strength on a regular basis. This list is also the standard that medical practitioners use to determine if your child is meeting motor milestones on time. If you are concerned that your baby is not developing on time, talk to your child's doctor.

CARDIOPULMONARY SYSTEM AND MOBILITY

Next, we are going to briefly review the development of the cardiopulmonary system. This includes the heart and the lungs. As you can imagine, there is a change in the heart's function when a baby is born and no longer relying on the mother's body through the umbilical cord.

At birth, the pressures change in the heart as the baby's circulation stabilizes. It is not uncommon for a newborn to have an irregular electrocardiogram (ECG) reading during this stabilization period. The heart muscle, heartbeat, and heart position are all in flux. Initially, the baby's heart is horizontal in the chest; it becomes more vertical as the lungs expand and take on their new role of providing oxygen to the body.

Reciprocally, the lungs start off with small airways because, until birth, the baby has not had to breathe on her own. As she ages and the demands for oxygen increase, these airways become bigger. Not only are the airways initially smaller, but they are also weaker and less efficient than those of adults. This can cause a few complications. One of these is greater resistance to airflow, causing increased work to breathe. Also, due to their small size, airways can easily be obstructed by foreign objects.[1]

The mechanics of the infant lung is significant as well. It is not unusual for a newborn to have irregular breathing, just as it is not unusual for her to have an irregular heartbeat. This includes periods of apnea (not breathing). Because they are new to breathing, babies' ribs are not in proper angular alignment to support it. This alignment of the ribs around the lungs develops as muscles get stronger.

A newborn's shoulders are also elevated in the beginning. This structural immaturity, coupled with the lack of control of the abdominal muscles, prevents complete stabilization of the ribs and effective use of the diaphragm to breathe. It is not until the baby learns to move her head and upper body against gravity that this system begins to mature and make breathing easier.[1] It is important for your baby to develop antigravity strength, not only for development, but also to allow her to breathe easier, without working so hard.

As discussed previously, we develop antigravity strength of the head and the upper body by lying on our stomachs. If you do not lie on your stomach in early childhood development, you cannot develop optimal strength necessary for breathing! Infants should develop this ability to move their heads and upper bodies, as well as to reach for things, while on the stomach by the first three to six months. In the second half of the first year, your baby is sitting up, crawling, and walking, which expands the lungs' capacity, increases the spaces between the ribs, strengthens the abdominal muscles, and aligns the diaphragm in the proper position to develop effective breathing.

Parents often tell me they do not place their baby on her stomach "because she cries." They are not alone. It is reported that 25 percent of parents never place their babies on their stomach, even to play.[4]

It stands to reason that a baby would cry when placed on her stomach if she is not accustomed to lying in that fashion.

First of all, because of a lack of muscle strength, the baby is not able to move as easily on her stomach and cannot see as well as she can on her back. Secondly, the pressure on her stomach and lungs from lying on them is an unaccustomed sensation. Remember that the baby's lungs have to expand to the back as well as the front, for the muscles of the ribs and back to become strong for breathing. Babies who consistently lie on their stomachs are much less likely to object to this position. It may be a process of getting your child used to stomach lying, but it is well worth it.

Physiological development occurs when a baby is given time to move around in her environment unrestricted. Motor development starts from the horizontal position in an environment that provides the room and security to just explore and move around. Furthermore, according to studies of infants and toddlers, children who seek out interaction and stimulation with their environment at an early age displayed higher levels of cognitive, academic, and neurophysiologic abilities later in life. Being mobile allows infants and toddlers the opportunity to develop better peripheral vision, as well as increasing awareness of activities that happen at a distance. There is a direct relationship between the amount of physical activity engaged in and whether a child will meet motor milestones on schedule. Additionally, research indicates that more physical activity early in life might prevent chronic illness and obesity later in life.[5]

In conclusion, normal development is designed to occur in a very specific fashion. This process cannot be rushed, nor can it occur if a baby is restricted or confined. It is normal for babies to develop at their own rate and to develop skills in their own time. That means it is also normal for any given child to acquire a skill earlier or later than what is considered "normal." As long as your baby is developing in the normal range, there is little reason to be alarmed. But remember, if a baby does not develop antigravity muscle strength by being placed in different positions (that is, on the stomach), it can complicate the normal physiologic process for developing the lungs and progressing with developmental milestone acquisition.

2

REFLEXES

The link to survival for all infants comes from the brainstem. This is the only part of the brain that functions properly at birth. The brainstem is responsible for breathing, body temperature, blood pressure, levels of arousal, and the fight-or-flight response of the autonomic nervous system. It receives sensory information from the environment and from inside the body, then links it to the cortex, the part of the brain responsible for movement. Because the infant is receiving a vast array of impulses from the environment after delivery, new nerve-cell branches are laid down in high numbers—an estimated 4.7 million every minute. Without interaction with the environment, brain maturation can be delayed or impaired.[2]

A reflex is an involuntary reaction or movement.[6] We are born equipped with them as both an immediate means for survival as well as an aid in development. Reflexes also originate in the brainstem. They exist to get us moving when our muscles are not quite coordinated or strong enough to get the job done. For instance, the symmetrical tonic neck reflex (STNR) prepares us for crawling on all fours by getting us up on our hands and knees. The Landau reflex helps increase the muscle tone of the back and neck so that when a baby is lying on his stomach, he can lift up his chest and reach for things. Besides the kinesthetic development, both of these reflexes also help a baby develop near and far vision, because he alternately focuses on things directly in front of him and objects off in the distance.

Each reflex has a parallel movement and development goal for the different sensory systems of the brain and body. And each occurs at a different time in development, creating a window of opportunity, if you will, to capitalize on its presence. Some reflexes only occur for a brief period of time; then they go away as they are integrated into the developing person, once no longer needed. Examples of these are the rooting reflex of the mouth and the grasp reflex of the hand, both designed specifically for newborns to seek food and hold onto safety. Others arise and continue to exist throughout our entire lives for protection. An example of this is the *protective extension reflex*, in which we put our hands out to catch ourselves if we fall.

If a reflex doesn't emerge when it is supposed to, problems can arise. These can include low muscle tone, muscle weakness, chronic body aches, poor endurance, and fatigue. If reflexes persist longer than they are intended to even more issues can arise, such as challenges with coordination, reading and writing difficulties, language and speech delays, disorganization, fidgeting, poor bladder control, and breathing difficulties.[2]

What can cause reflexes to not behave as they are intended to? Stress of the mother and/or baby during pregnancy, breech birth, birth trauma, caesarean birth, and induced birth are a few surrounding the birthing process itself. During infancy, reflexes can be hampered by lack of enough proper movement, being overly encumbered in walkers, jumpers, or being left for long periods of time in car seats, bouncers, or cribs. Illness, trauma, injury, chronic stress, environmental toxins, complications with vaccinations, as well as dietary imbalances or sensitivities are other potential issues that may cause reflexes to not perform as designed.[2] Furthermore, many reflexes can only be accessed from the prone position. In other words, they require that the baby be placed on his stomach to utilize them.

Adults can suffer from reflexes not properly integrated during childhood. Many conditions, from back pain to anxiety, are the result of undeveloped or *unintegrated* reflexes that persist into adulthood.[2] For example, the spinal galant reflex assists the baby in moving down the birth canal during delivery. It is displayed when the area next to the spine is touched at the waist level, resulting in the hips turning toward that side. It should disappear three to six months after delivery. Children born by cesarean section (C-section) often have this reflex persisting. The result is that the child—and later on, the adult—learns to fix the hips to prevent movement when this area of the back is touched by the back of a chair, a belt worn on the pants, etc. This strain against the persistent reflex results in back pain. For children who display the spinal galant reflex, fidgeting in school is also common, because the back is being touched and the reflex stimulated when they are sitting at their desks.

In the event of a stroke or brain injury, sometimes adults revert back to the survival mode of the brainstem and have to relearn the many functions of the body. During this process, reflexes often reemerge and must be redeveloped or reintegrated for the person to move forward with recovery.

There are various methods of treating un-integrated reflexes, including yoga, postural restoration, and rhythmic movement training. However, the best form of treatment is prevention. Allowing infants to move about freely in their environment, along with sufficient physical contact from their caregivers—rocking, hugging, gentle grooming, etc.—allows the process to happen naturally.

3

SUDDEN INFANT DEATH SYNDROME—SIDS

SIDS is the primary concern for the majority of the parents with whom I speak. Certainly, nothing can be more frightening than the prospect of your child dying in its sleep from no apparent cause. However, I have found that very few people have accurate information about SIDS and are therefore in a state of reaction to the bits and pieces they hear in the media, on the Internet, and from people around them. In most cases, it is the temptation to draw conclusions from only part of the information that is fueling the way parents take care of their babies. As a pediatric physical therapist, I spend every day educating the parents and caregivers of my patients, often dispensing the same professional advice over and over regarding sleeping position. In this chapter, we are going to define sudden infant death syndrome and discuss the leading theories for what may be causing it.

SIDS is defined as the sudden, unexplained death of an infant younger than one year old, which remains unknown after an autopsy, death-scene investigation, and review of medical history. It is also known as crib death and cot death. According to the *National Vital Statistics Reports* published by the Centers for Disease Control and Prevention (CDC) for 2009, SIDS is the third leading cause of infant mortality in the United States.[7] Most SIDS deaths happen when babies are between two and four months old. African American babies are more than twice as likely to die of SIDS as white babies, and American Indian/

Alaskan Native babies are nearly three times as likely to die of SIDS as white babies.[8]

Many theories have arisen over the years in the effort to explain the cause of crib death. More recently, the focus has been on certain areas of the brain and certain heart defects. It is possible that there is not one singular cause of unexplained infant death, but many.

The leading theory denoted in the policy statement from the American Academy of Pediatrics states that these babies may have a "maldeveloped or delay in maturation of the brainstem neural network that is responsible for arousal and affects the physiologic responses to life-threatening challenges during sleep."[9] What that means is if the brainstem is not working correctly, for whatever reason, it can affect the baby's ability to keep himself alive while asleep.

Information in the brain is sent to other areas of the body and brain through naturally occurring chemicals messengers called neurotransmitters. Serotonin is one of these chemical messengers that work in the brainstem. There are receptor sites—kind of like loading docks—that receive the chemical message, which then causes the brain or the body to respond in one way or the other.

According to WebMD Health News published on February 2, 2010, researcher Hannah Kinney, MD, professor of pathology at Harvard Medical School and neuropathologist, along with her colleagues, studied thirty-five infants who died of SIDS. These babies were found to have 26 percent lower serotonin levels than babies who had died of known causes. The study reported that there was a lower level of "binding to the receptors that utilize serotonin in the brainstem." Dr. Kinney suggested that serotonin levels and the level of arousal are important in SIDS. She also pointed out in this study that serotonin may be a significant factor, but possibly not the only chemical messenger involved.[10]

Another study, published in 1998, cited increased levels of serotonin found in adult subjects who died of heart failure. It stated, "We conclude that serotonin is involved in the syndrome of heart failure both directly and indirectly through its action on cardiac contractility, heart rate, preload and afterload."[11] In other words, serotonin acts on the cardiovascular system (heart, veins and arteries) in addition to working in the brain. It makes blood vessels constrict or become narrow.[6] In this instance, high levels of serotonin in the blood were associated with heart failure.

Much research has been done in recent years pointing to heart problems as the culprit for SIDS. The focus is on the conduction system of the heart, which keeps it beating normally. This system is called the Bundle of His (named for Swiss cardiologist, Wilhelm His, Jr.) or the atrioventricular (AV) bundle (see fig. 1). It is the control center that coordinates the four chambers of the heart as they fill with blood and pump it out in a rhythmic fashion. Abnormalities in this system would cause the heart to beat erratically and, therefore, not be able to function as the pump it is designed to. If the heart is damaged in one part of the muscle, the cardiac cycle can become uncoordinated and chaotic, which can become fatal if not treated immediately.[12]

Figure 1: Bundle of His

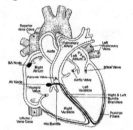

A study conducted in 1985 examined the hearts of twenty-three infants, fifteen who died of SIDS and eight of known causes. An abnormality in the left side of the AV bundle was found in eight of the fifteen SIDS hearts. This led the researchers to conclude the bundle of His might also be a factor in SIDS.[13]

Another study performed in 1976 analyzed fifty infant hearts on autopsy. Twenty-six of these were said to be SIDS cases and twenty-four were from known causes of death. When comparing the two groups, abnormalities in the heart tissue were almost identical in both groups of infants. Hemorrhage in or around the conduction system of the heart was found in 27 percent of SIDS babies and 29 percent of those determined to have an explained death.[14] These results bring to question whether the twenty-six babies who were diagnosed with SIDS were actually misdiagnosed heart defects.

In 2008, Dr. Andrew Ewer, senior clinical research fellow in the Department of Pediatrics and Child Health at the University of Birmingham in the UK, reported that congenital heart disease is the most common group of congenital malformations in newborns. He wrote, "It contributes to 3% of all infant mortality and 46% of deaths from congenital malformations, with most deaths occurring in the first year of life."[15] Remember that SIDS also occurs, by definition, in the first year of life.

Another focus area has been on what is considered fatal arrhythmias from occult long QT syndrome. Below is the picture of a normal heartbeat (see fig. 2). Each letter represents something occurring in the heart in one of the four chambers that reside there. The heart experiences a cyclical filling and emptying of these chambers through contracting and relaxing. This process acts to pump blood throughout the body.

Figure 2: Heartbeat

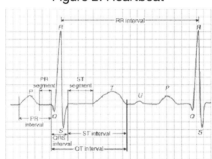

The QT segment represents the time for electrical activation (contracting) and inactivation (relaxing) of the ventricles in the heart's lower chambers. During the QRS, the ventricles are contracting and pushing blood out. And during T, they are recovering their energy to get ready to contract again, once filled with blood. If this process of contracting and relaxing takes longer than usual, a heart rhythm disorder can potentially occur resulting in fast, chaotic heartbeats. This is called *long QT syndrome* (LQTS) and is a known cause of sudden death. At the 2005 annual meeting of the Heart Rhythm Society, Marianne

Arnestad, MD, reported that SIDS cases can be explained 12-15 percent of the time as caused by long QT syndrome.[16]

A long QT segment is one that shows up longer on the electrocardiogram (ECG) than what is considered normal, but it varies with individual heart rates. According to a Mayo Clinic article on long QT syndrome, "You can be born with a genetic mutation that puts you at risk for long QT syndrome."[17] In addition, there are more than fifty medications that can actually *cause* long QT syndrome. These include antihistamines, decongestants, diuretics, antibiotics, cholesterol-lowering medications, and some for diabetes.[18]

There is good news in all of this! These heart-related SIDS deaths are preventable through early identification of children with long QT syndrome, who are treated right away. Treatment options include medications, medical devices, and surgical intervention, which result in a much lower rate of illness and death. Mayo Clinic included in the article the symptoms of long QT syndrome. Fainting is the most common sign of this condition. Linked to these fainting spells is anger, excitability, fear, or exertion, which changes the way the heart beats. Seizures are another sign of long QT syndrome. Signs and symptoms of inherited long QT syndrome may start as early as the first month of life or as late as middle age. Most people have their first episode by the age of forty, and most deaths from this condition occur between the ages of eleven and thirty years old. However, it reports that long QT symptoms rarely occur during sleep or arousal from sleep.[17]

SSRIs and SIDS

In a related topic, we are going to take a brief look at taking antidepressants during pregnancy. Some antidepressants work by affecting serotonin in the body. These are referred to collectively as *selective serotonin reuptake inhibitors* or SSRIs. Since the current leading theory for SIDS focuses on the level of serotonin in infants, this area merits discussion.

A study was published in November 2009 in which 38,602 Norwegian children were monitored through the first year of life. Of these children, 197 were born to mothers who used antidepressants throughout pregnancy, 820 stopped using antidepressants before pregnancy, and 543 used them only at certain points during the pregnancy. Seventy-one percent used an SSRI such as Prozac or Paxil. It was not clarified how soon before pregnancy those who stopped taking the medication actually discontinued use.

Elevated rates of congenital heart defects, respiratory distress, feeding problems, and irritability of the baby were reported in both groups of mothers who took antidepressants during pregnancy as well as those who stopped taking them before pregnancy. The researchers suggested this to be a result of the depression itself and its effects on the body of the mother. The possibility was also raised that antidepressants could still act upon the fetus early in the pregnancy due to the physiological effects of the drug as it was leaving the mother's system.[19]

This study raises the question of the genetic predisposition of serotonin levels passed from mother to baby. If the mother struggles with depression and must therefore rely on antidepressant medications that affect serotonin, is the baby's level of serotonin genetically altered?

Taking medication at all presents a health risk during pregnancy. In particular, some of the common SSRIs have been associated with newborn complications. Celexa, Paxil, and Zoloft for example, have been associated with a variety of problems, which might include a rare but serious newborn lung problem called *persistent pulmonary hypertension of the newborn* (PPHN), septal heart defects (holes in the heart), birth defects that affect the brain and skull, birth defects that affect the sutures of the skull, and a birth defect that affects the abdominal organs. Although these conditions are said to be rare or the risks low, they still constitute a risk to the baby of a mother who takes antidepressants during pregnancy.[20]

As depression itself can affect a woman during pregnancy, it is up to the mother and the doctor's discretion as to the benefit of discontinuing antidepressants. In some cases, the mother could pose a risk to herself and her baby if she stops taking the medication. A mother may turn to alcohol or drugs during the pregnancy to cope with depression or may stop taking care of herself and, in turn, the unborn baby. It is a difficult decision to make at best, and one best left to the individual case of mother and doctor.[20]

From my perspective, it would be helpful to know if any of these mothers in this study had babies die unexpectedly. This information was not included, but would be very valuable. This connection may be on the horizon or a study currently underway. But, after an extensive search, I have yet to find it.

An invaluable resource for more information can be found at www.sids-network.org, an online forum where people can write in questions about their individual cases and receive answers from the leading medical experts in the field of sudden infant death syndrome. You may find the SIDS Network helpful if you still have questions.

Obviously, the fear of SIDS has had a profound impact on the way parents care for their infants. It is possible that there may not be a single cause of sudden infant death syndrome, but rather, many different causes. As researchers are learning more by investigating infants who died unexpectedly, we are possibly getting closer to explaining most if not all sudden infant deaths.

4

SCREENING

Screening is a procedure, test, or examination that can identify the signs and symptoms of a disorder. If those signs and symptoms are detected, further testing will be done to determine if the condition exists. Screening newborns is on the rise in North America and abroad with the advent of current medical technology. With these processes, certain abnormalities in the body can be discovered and treated sooner, thus saving lives. As researchers are working diligently to find the true causes of sudden infant death syndrome, new doors are opening for doctors in knowing what to screen for. Every state in the United States has regulations and requirements for newborn screening. Some states test for more than fifty-four disorders, whereas others test for less than twenty-nine.[21] Currently, the tools available for screening include ultrasound, ECG, pulse oximetry, and blood tests.

ULTRASOUND

First marketed for use in obstetrics in 1983, ultrasound was not routinely used during pregnancy until the 1990s. The benefit of ultrasound is that fetal malformation can usually be detected before twenty weeks of pregnancy. Some common examples of these abnormalities are hydrocephalus, orthopedic disorders, and spina bifida. Conditions such as cleft lip and cleft palate and congenital cardiac abnormalities are more readily diagnosed and at an earlier gestational age with the development of the most recent equipment. Typically, an ultrasound is performed at seven weeks' gestation to confirm pregnancy, rule out ectopic pregnancy, confirm cardiac pulse, and measure the length of the baby to determine gestational age.

At eighteen to twenty weeks' gestation, doctors are mainly looking for congenital malformations. Fetal anatomy, multiple pregnancies, confirmation of due date, and growth of the baby can also be assessed, plus placental position determined.

Further scans may be necessary if abnormalities are suspected, and some centers will do blood-test biochemical screening as well. This type of screening has been monumental in detecting potentially fatal conditions in infants.[22]

Congenital heart defects occur in eight of every one thousand newborns, making them the most common birth defect. Although many heart defects do not require medical intervention, the more complex they are, the more likely they are to require treatment soon after the baby is born. Two heart defects commonly detected by ultrasound are holes in the heart (septal defects) and tetralogy of Fallot.

The *septum* is the wall that separates the four chambers of the heart. One side of the heart contains blood that is rich in oxygen from the lungs, which is then pumped throughout the body. The other side of the heart contains oxygen-poor blood that it has received from the body and will pump to the lungs to become oxygenated. If there is a septal defect, or hole in the heart, the blood with oxygen and the blood without mix, and poorly oxygenated blood can be pumped into the body. The body needs fully oxygenated blood to function.[23]

The most common, complex congenital heart defect is tetralogy of Fallot (TOF). It is actually a combination of four abnormalities:

- hardening of the heart valve that leads to the lungs (pulmonary valve stenosis),
- a large septal heart defect (ventricular septal defect-VSD),

- an abnormal position of the valve that directs oxygenated blood to the body (aorta), and
- right-sided heart-muscle thickening in the lower chamber (ventricle hypertrophy), due to the heart working harder than normal.

When TOF is detected by ultrasound, open-heart surgery typically takes place soon after birth.[23]

In the last twenty years, technology has improved the detection and treatment of congenital heart defects, ensuring that these infants can survive into adulthood. Currently, it is estimated that one million adults are living with congenital heart defects in the United States.[23]

ECG

In 2008, a group of computer scientists, molecular biologists, and cardiologists at the University of Pavia in Italy screened 45,000 babies for a heart rhythm disorder using ECG and then evaluated the costs and benefits of screening. An electrocardiogram or ECG is a painless and noninvasive way to record the electrical activity of the heart. It works by putting *leads* (they look like stickers) on the chest that send information to a machine regarding how the heart is beating. ECG is also inexpensive and accurate in testing the heart for electrical conduction abnormalities. If you recall, the bundle of His is the conduction system of the heart. The conclusion of the study was that a significant number of sudden deaths could be prevented if ECG was part of the neonatal screening process.[24]

Remember that long QT syndrome is also detectable through ECG. Dr. Marianne Arnestad strongly recommended at the annual meeting of the Heart Rhythm Society that doctors screen *all neonates* for prolonged QT using ECG, with follow-up genetic testing for those infants suspected of having it. If you have a family member who has long QT syndrome or who has died from this condition, it would be very wise to have your baby screened.[16]

PULSE OXIMETRY

Things to look for in the future include one proposed study in the United Kingdom in which researchers will evaluate the effectiveness of using pulse oximetry as a screening test for congenital heart disease in newborn babies.[15] Pulse oximetry is a noninvasive diagnostic test used for measuring the amount of oxygen in the blood. It works by putting a plastic device on the end of your finger that sends information to a machine. The amount of oxygen in your blood is indicative of whether your heart and lungs are working properly. Non-invasive screening tests are preferred by hospitals and insurance companies for several reasons with cost being at the top of the list.

BLOOD TESTS

Routine newborn screening programs currently exist for metabolic, endocrine, and hematologic disorders. These are discovered through a blood test, which involves taking a small vile of blood from the infant and testing it for known abnormalities. It is estimated that six babies are born every day in the United States with one of these disorders, but go undetected because they are not screened. This is unfortunate, because most of these types of disorders are treatable through dietary restrictions. And, it is estimated that 5 percent of SIDS cases are actually undiagnosed metabolic disorders.[25]

One way to have your baby screened for something specific is to ask your child's doctor. He or she can order a metabolic screen, an ECG, or other test for your newborn. Alternatively, screening agencies exist throughout the United States where you can bring your baby for an in-depth screen or mail a vile of your baby's blood to be tested. These agencies operate by charging either a fee per screening test or a flat fee for a certain number of screens.

If you choose to go the agency route, do so with caution. It is recommended that you verify the integrity of the organization through the local and national regulation agencies to safeguard yourself and your newborn.

In conclusion, the medical community is embarking on an ongoing, massive research journey to prevent SIDS, which includes the use of screening tools. Detecting disorders and treating them right away is saving lives. But understand that *there is no full-proof screening test.* All tests come with the caveat that some cases could be missed on the one hand, and on the other, some babies could receive a diagnosis when they do not actually have a problem.

In addition, the cost of screening newborns may be considered an excessive expenditure by some hospitals and some insurance carriers. For the rest of us, there is no cost greater than losing a child. So, I encourage you to get as much information as you can for you and your baby. What you know could save your newborn's life.

5

BACK TO SLEEP PROGRAM

In 1992, the release of the SIDS reports in Europe and Australia prompted the American Academy of Pediatrics (AAP) to begin recommending placing babies on their backs to sleep. A task force from the United States then began a study regarding sleep position and SIDS. The study, led by the National Institute of Child Health and Human Development, was composed of a national sampling to determine if parents were adhering to the recommendation to place infants on their back to sleep.[9]

The Back to Sleep campaign was launched in 1994. The effort was under the direction of the National Institute of Child Health and Human Development, a division of the National Institutes of Health (NIH). The program was backed by the US Public Health Service, the AAP, the SIDS Alliance, and the Association of SIDS and Infant Mortality Program. Along with the AAP in the United States, New Zealand, Tasmania, the United Kingdom, Australia, Denmark, Norway, Sweden, and the Netherlands began to recommend back sleeping as well.[9]

Multiple studies that followed in the United States and abroad regarding sleep position, bed sharing, sleep surface, and parental smoking habits revealed that in Europe and North America, the SIDS rate in January is double that of the summer months, with the majority occurring from October through April. In New Zealand, the majority of babies who died were found lying on their stomachs on sheepskin. In Australia, babies died when

33

face down on soft, crib mattresses filled with natural fibers like Ti tree bark. Also, there was a high incidence of babies found face down on a pillow or soft mattress with the nose and mouth covered by bedding.[9]

The European Concerted Action on SIDS study found 77 percent of SIDS cases involved bed sharing with a mother who smoked. Additionally, 62 percent of babies had their heads covered and were lying on their stomachs.[26]

An increased risk of SIDS was found when there were multiple bed sharers, especially when the bed sharers were other children. There was also an increased risk of infant death with parents using alcohol or drugs or when they were overly tired and shared a bed with an infant.[9]

In 2005, preliminary data reported the SIDS rate had decreased by 53 percent from 1994 to 2003, since the inception of The Back to Sleep campaign.[9]

Figure 3: Back to Sleep Chart

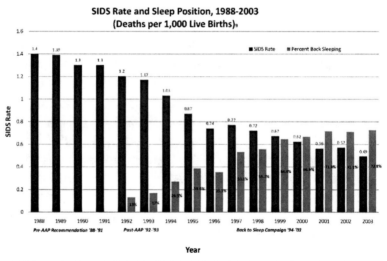

The data states 1.2 SIDS deaths per 1,000 live births occurred in 1992, whereas 0.56 SIDS deaths per 1,000 live births were reported in 2001. The rate in 2002 did not change from the previous year. In addition, the infant rate of death from all causes decreased by 27 percent in the same time period. Interestingly, from 1992-2001, it is reported that the rate of other causes of sudden unexpected infant death increased dramatically indicating that infant deaths previously classified as SIDS are now being diagnosed as the result of other causes. The AAP policy statement reveals that because of this change in infant mortality diagnostics, the "true SIDS rate" since 1999 may remain the same[9].

If you were to review the task force's recommendations, you would find a total of fourteen recommendations. The first refers to actual sleep position, recommending that each sleep should occur on the back. As you continue down the list, you will see the importance of firm bedding, removing soft, loose items from the sleeping area. It is recommended not to smoke around a baby or share a sleeping environment with the baby, avoid overheating, etc. It is not until you get to the end of the list that issues like development, head shape, prolonged car seat use, etc., arise. Before I began research for this book, I would have told you with certainty that there was only one recommendation and it was to place your baby on the back to sleep. Personally, I was unaware of the other thirteen recommendations, and I suspect many others are not either.

Unfortunately, the one recommendation that has received the most press is the message of "Only place your baby on the back to sleep." This translates to most people as "Never place your baby on his stomach." Also missed is the recommendation to avoid prolonged use of car seats and bouncers, which is occurring at epidemic numbers today. Among the recommendations is to avoid plagiocephaly. How many people even know what "plagiocephaly" is? (We will discuss plagiocephaly (flattening of the head) in detail in an upcoming chapter.) More important, how many people would read the entire list?

According to the Center for Disease Control and Prevention (CDC), an infant sleeping on a soft surface *and* lying on his stomach was at a far greater risk of SIDS than just lying on his stomach or just lying on a soft surface. In this report, soft bedding, independent of sleep position, posed 5 times the risk of SIDS than firm bedding, whereas sleeping on the stomach posed a lower 2.4 times the risk. But, infants lying are on their stomachs *and* on soft bedding were at 21 times the risk of SIDS as infants who slept on their back on firm bedding.[27] Therefore, it is not as important which position your child is lying in, but rather *what* he is laying on. Lying on the stomach on a firm surface has one of the lowest risk factors of SIDS, yet the majority of people do not place their babies on the stomach—sometimes ever—because of the Back to Sleep program and the belief that it will prevent SIDS.

The recommendations warn against soft mattresses, soft bedding, soft items like stuffed animals in the bed, soft "pillow-like" bumper pads, etc. With the above statistic, it stands to reason that the most important message should be to avoid soft bedding and soft items in the bed. Consider an adult mattress: it is designed for comfort for an adult. But for an infant, a pillow top or cushy mattress can be very hazardous, because newborns lack ample muscle strength to move about. Thus, infants should not be allowed to sleep in their parents' bed for the simple fact that the mattress is too soft.

The task force also cited that an infant sleeping on a couch or sofa is at a much higher risk for SIDS than sleeping in a crib or on another hard surface. The experts say they don't know why this is, but warns that it is extremely dangerous.[9] Again, it can be concluded, the soft material poses the greater threat, regardless of which position the baby is sleeping in.

The issue of bed sharing is a red flag. It is common to believe that if the baby sleeps with one or both parents, he will be safe. The NICHD reports that there is no scientific proof that bed sharing between an adult and a child reduces SIDS. In fact, numerous studies have concluded that a baby sleeping with either the mother alone or both parents was associated with *an increased* risk of SIDS.[27]

We can surmise there are two possible reasons for this. One, the bed of the parent is too soft; and two, there is a higher risk of suffocation due to the parent rolling over on the child while asleep. The latter actually refers to accidental death and, by definition, cannot be SIDS, whose cause is unknown. Another recommendation states you should not sleep with an infant if you are excessively tired or using medications that alter your alertness. By definition, a new parent *is* excessively tired!

Sleeping with other children seems to threaten an even higher risk for SIDS. The CDC reports that infants who died of SIDS were 5.4 times more likely to have shared a bed with other children. If you recall, African American babies are more than twice as likely to die of SIDS as white babies. According to CDC director Dr. Julie Gerberding, families of this origin "need to know they should avoid putting an infant to sleep with other children."[27] In an attempt to reduce this racial disparity, a large group of African American organizations including the Congress of National Black Churches, the National Black Child Development Institute, the National Coalition of 100 Black Women, to name a few, launched an educational outreach program to reduce the number of SIDS of African American babies.[27]

In conclusion, with the launch of the Back to Sleep program, the main focus has been the placement of your baby on his or her back to sleep to prevent SIDS. The majority of parents I talk with in my practice are not aware of the other recommendations by the AAP for safe sleeping habits—as I would guess most people are not. It is clear that the emphasis has been placed in the wrong area. Soft bedding, soft mattresses, and soft items in the crib are a far greater concern for a baby's health, with bed sharing close behind. However, this raises an even bigger question. Is it SIDS or accidental suffocation that is to blame in the instance of a baby's face being covered? Is it correct to call it SIDS when a mother accidently rolls over on top of her infant while sleeping? We will discuss this as well as the other issues associated with the Back to Sleep Program in the next few chapters.

The take-home message is this:

- *Do NOT* put your baby on soft bedding to sleep, especially on his stomach.
- *Do NOT* put your baby to sleep on a couch or armchair.

- *Do NOT* allow your baby to share a bed with you, other adults, or other children—especially with other children!

These are the highest risk factors for SIDS and the most important guidelines for you to follow.

6

Back to Sleep and SIDS

It is important to realize the interrelationship between the Back to Sleep program and SIDS. Studies tell us that certain malformations in the brain or heart can be the cause of sudden infant death. The leading theory points to serotonin. Lower levels of serotonin were found in babies who died with a diagnosis of SIDS. What does this mean?

In a normal situation, if a baby is face down on a soft surface, say a comforter, and is re-breathing the same air, her internal oxygen balance will be lower than what she needs; so, the brainstem will sound an alarm or an internal trigger, signaling the baby to respond by changing positions, turning her head, rolling over, or some other mean of getting a better supply of oxygen. *If a baby has a lower level of serotonin, that alarm may not sound,* that internal trigger will not cause the baby to adapt to the change, and she may not adjust her position to get a better supply of oxygen. The result could be that she expires.

Similarly, if she is lying on her back and a stuffed animal falls across her face causing her to re-breathe the same air, the result would be the same. This situation is referred to as *positional asphyxia*, but is still diagnosed as SIDS in many cases. The rationale is that the baby has some *internal* defect that prevents her from responding to a life-threatening situation in her environment.

There are some very fuzzy and gray lines when you look at suffocation, asphyxia, and SIDS. Suffocation is defined as death caused by obstruction of the airways. Suffocation could occur if a baby chokes on a small toy or is trapped underneath another child and cannot breathe. Asphyxia is an inadequate intake of oxygen and exhalation of carbon dioxide.[28] This could occur if a baby is face down on a pillow. These terms are very similar and the external circumstances would be the only indicator of what actually happened. Ultimately, the end result would be the same, making the final diagnosis key. Suffocation? Asphyxia? SIDS?

Scripps Howard News Service wondered the same thing and so launched a nine-month investigation in 2007. They studied unexpected infant deaths from all over the country. The conclusion was that "most of these babies are suffocating in completely avoidable accidents," and that "most coroners are not following the methods of investigation recommended by the CDC, prompting them to instead rely on often incorrect diagnoses of SIDS."[29]

The investigation cited unsafe sleeping environments as the most common reason for infant death. The researchers went on to say that it is rare for a baby to die while sleeping alone in a crib. Dr. Andrea Minyard, the Florida state medical examiner, reported, "It is far more common for a child to die of asphyxiation than to die of SIDS. Most of the time, it is parent overlay or unsafe and excessive bedding."[29]

The study identified eleven coroners who were using federally recommended best practices when examining infant death. These eleven cited approximately 71 percent of infant deaths in their jurisdictions were accidental suffocations, not SIDS. Three common elements were found with all eleven officials:

The corners' investigators, who were trained in forensic methods, were dispatched to the scene instead of relying on the police report;

The investigators utilized the CDC's Sudden Unexplained Infant Death Investigation protocol to guide the investigation;

The coroners reported their findings to the local child death review team.

The Scripps investigation found that states with both local and statewide child death review boards are identifying more than twice as many suffocations than states with little or no review. These eleven coroners believe the SIDS diagnosis is being overused.[29]

Tom Haynes, acting coroner in Omaha, claimed, "If the family doesn't admit to lying on top of the child during sleep, something I've never known to happen, then we have no choice but to call it SIDS."[29]

Dr. John McGoff, coroner for Indianapolis through 2004, was quoted saying, "As a coroner, you don't want to look into the face of a grandmother or father or mother who rolled over and smothered a child. There is no way to console them. But, without that knowledge, there's no prevention."[29]

Two-thirds of the forty-one sudden infant deaths examined by the Florida state medical examiner, Dr. Andrea Minyard, were accidental asphyxiations. She determined, "These infants die because they are accidentally smothered by their parents or other children who sleep with them or because they are placed in dangerous overstuffed sofas or heavily blanketed adult beds."[29]

Dr. John Carroll of the Johns Hopkins Children's Center reported, "It is true that the CPSC (Consumer Product Safety Commission) reported that some deaths diagnosed as SIDS were likely due to suffocation caused by unsafe crib and bedding materials, and I suspect they are right."[28] In an article published January 26, 2009, in *Pediatrics*, the CDC reported, "Infant deaths related to suffocation and strangulation in bed have *quadrupled* in the last two decades."[30]

That seems to be a chilling statistic, but if we look back at the chart presented in the chapter on the Back to Sleep program, the last two decades were precisely the period that we supposedly had the greatest decrease in SIDS. It is possible we were simply trading diagnoses; moreover, previous reports of SIDS may not have been unexplained deaths at all, but merely misdiagnosed. Also, consider this: screening by ultrasound arrived in full force in the early 1990s and has become key in detecting congenital defects. Again, this is precisely the time that the rate of SIDS began its major decline. Perhaps it is not the rate of sudden infant death syndrome that is decreasing; rather we are just able to explain more of the deaths with current technology. Remember, SIDS should be given as a diagnosis when the death remains unknown after all other factors have been eliminated through autopsy, death scene investigation, and a review of medical history.

INFANT MORTALITY

So, what is the overall rate of infant mortality in the United States? Based on the latest statistics from the CDC, the current estimate for 2010 is 6.14 deaths per 1,000 children before their first birthday.[31] That is a slight decline from the rate in 2000, which was 6.86 deaths per 1,000 children.[32] The report indicates that there was not a change in infant mortality from 2000-2005.[32] But there has been a significant decline from the previous decades: in 1990, the rate was 9.2 per 1,000 births, and in 1980, it was 12.5 per 1,000 births.[33] This indicates that coupled with the SIDS rate dropping, so has the overall infant mortality rate in the United States.

The leading cause of infant death is congenital defects—birth defects—which occur during fetal development in the womb. Approximately 5,500 babies died in 2005 from congenital defects such as heart defects. Preterm birth and low-weight birth are the second highest causes of infant death, with 4,698 in 2005. A preterm birth is one that occurs before thirty-seven weeks of pregnancy.[34] Statistics show that preterm birth is on the rise with a 9 percent increase from 2000-2005. In 2005, 68.5 percent of all infant deaths were preterm infants with 36.5 percent of these directly related to preterm complications.

In the United States, approximately two-thirds of infant deaths occur in the baby's first month of life due most often to problems with the pregnancy or health problems of the baby, including birth defects. One-third of infant deaths that occur after the first month are influenced by social and environmental issues like cigarette smoke in the home.[33]

Sudden infant death syndrome is considered the *third* leading cause of infant death and accounted for approximately

2,200 infants in 2005.[34] Harvard Medical School professor and neuropathologist Hannah Kinney, MD, was quoted early in 2010 in *USA Today* saying, "The Back to Sleep campaign, begun in 1994, helped to cut SIDS deaths in half, although deaths have not declined further in the past decade."[35]

To conclude, if an infant is in an unsafe situation, the risk for sudden death is higher, regardless of any other factor. For instance, if a baby is asleep in a crib with a poorly fitted mattress, she can roll down between the mattress and the edge of the crib and get trapped. If she is asleep in an adult bed and the parent or another child rolls over on the baby, she can be smothered. If a baby is lying face down on a pillow or soft surface and cannot pull herself out of that position due to inadequate muscle strength, she can asphyxiate.

If you recall from the joint SIDS study conducted from 1992-1994 by the various countries, most babies found dead were in unsafe situations. The risk of SIDS with soft bedding material was independent of sleep position. The point here is if you really want to reduce the risk of sudden infant death, regardless of what the diagnosis, place your baby only in a safe situation to sleep. Research tells us this is alone, in a crib or bassinet, with a properly fitted, firm mattress, devoid of soft items. Sleep position is secondary to the safety of the sleep environment.

There is no question that the Back to Sleep campaign has saved many babies' lives by educating parents on the dangers of co-sleeping and soft bedding. I applaud the efforts of the task force and the coalition who have spent many years attempting to tackle the issue of SIDS. Much greatly needed research has come out of the process, which will likely save many more babies' lives.

It is essential that you understand the full picture of SIDS, screening, and the Back to Sleep campaign in order to best care for your infant. It is the misunderstanding of information that is drastically changing the way we care for our infants. As a result, certain infant diagnoses are on the rise. We will explore some of these problems that were born out of the SIDS-Back to Sleep Era.

7

TORTICOLLIS AND PLAGIOCEPHALY

Since the inception of the Back to Sleep program, the incidence of *torticollis* has increased by 84 percent. Reports indicate it occurs in one in three hundred infants.[36] Sometimes called wryneck, torticollis is the abnormal shortening of the muscles on one or both sides of the neck, causing the head to lean to one side. When this occurs, the baby often adopts a favored lying position with the head always turned to the same side. Subsequently, facial or skull deformities can occur, as well as deficits in the visual field. This muscle imbalance can cause scoliosis of the neck and result in abnormal movement patterns as well.

Most often, the *sternocleidomastiod* muscle, or SCM, is involved.[36] This is the muscle that attaches behind your ear and extends to your collarbone and sternum. The job of this muscle is to rotate the head to the opposite direction and to side-flex or bend your head to the same side. So, your left SCM bends your head to the left and rotates your head to the right, and your right SCM does the opposite, bending your head to the right and rotating it left. Another pair of muscles that can be involved are the trapezius muscles, which are attached to the back of your head and extend down to about the middle of your back. This muscle bends the head to one side if just one of them contracts and bends the head back if acting together. There are a few more deep, neck muscles whose job is to bend the head to the side, which can also be affected, such as the scalene muscles.

One of the most common causes of torticollis is the position a baby lies in most of the time. When a baby is lying on his back, the pull of gravity causes the head to turn to one side until there is adequate strength to hold the head in midline. If the baby favors lying with the head turned to one side a disproportionate amount of time, the muscles of that side will shorten, thus restricting rotation to the other side.

To give an example, if you put a cast on your arm with the elbow bent for six weeks, when the cast is removed, the muscles will be shortened on the front of the elbow and lengthened on the back. The shortened muscles will be uncomfortable to stretch out. Reciprocally, the lengthened muscles become weak.

Similarly, if the neck muscles are shortened on one side, it will be uncomfortable for the baby to rotate his head to the other side. In addition, the muscles on the other side will be overstretched and weak, compounding the problem and reinforcing the favored position.

The incidence of torticollis is increasing since the start of the Back to Sleep program, because parents are allowing babies to spend a disproportionate amount of time on their backs.[36] In addition, babies are spending very little time on their stomachs or sides and therefore are not developing balanced muscle strength of the neck and back.

Other causes for this shortening of neck muscles are from prenatal constraint, trauma at birth, or from a spasmodic condition. Prenatal constraint is typically due to limited space in the womb in the case of multiple births, forcing the baby to cock his head to one side during the final weeks of gestation. In addition, if the baby is big or the mother is small, this fetal crowding can also occur. In these cases, the limitation is usually detected when the baby is first born. The youngest babies being seen in the clinic with a shortened SCM are likely due to their position in the womb.

A few babies referred to our clinic had broken their collarbones during birth and thus developed torticollis. It was likely to have occurred when the muscles around the break healed, burdening one side with scar tissue, and thus shortening as the scar tissue contracted. A break makes it painful for the baby to move, so he probably won't, attributing to the shortening.

Shortened neck muscles can develop with babies who have frequent stomach upset or colic. Just as they don't want to move a painful, broken collarbone, babies will also lean away from a painful stomach. These babies often lean to one side and develop torticollis from being in this favored position more often than not.

Torticollis can also be spasmodic. It is unknown why this occurs, but it can cause a palpable knot in the SCM with

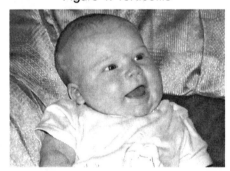

Figure 4: Torticollis

continuous contraction of this muscle. This occurs in 28-47 percent of babies with this diagnosis.[36] The leading theories suggest the baby was crowded in the womb (as with multiple births), muscle trauma during delivery, or a congenital abnormality.

The knot feels like an olive in the muscle belly when you rub your finger over it. Sometimes, it is large enough to see. It is the muscle spasm that makes spasmodic torticollis different from positional torticollis, in which the muscles are just shortened. The spasm causes the head to tilt. In positional torticollis, the consistent head tilt causes the muscles to shorten.

Children with eye muscle problems may turn or tilt their head to get a clear view of the world. These cases will present with no muscle tightness in the neck on evaluation, but have a head tilt to one side. This condition is called ocular torticollis.[36] Babies with this problem most often tilt their head away from the side of the affected eye. So, if the right eye is involved, they will side-bend to the left. When you cover the affected eye, the baby straightens his head. A referral to an eye doctor is the next step for these children. In most cases, the superior oblique muscle of the eye is involved and requires surgical correction.[37]

In addition to torticollis, the incidence of plagiocephaly has increased by 48 percent since the introduction of the Back to Sleep Program.[4] Plagiocephaly means a misshapen head, with the Greek root of the word meaning oblique head. There are three very different causes of plagiocephaly or misshapen head. The first involves abnormalities in the brain itself, which causes it to grow in unusual directions, affecting the shape of the skull. The second occurs when there is premature closing or fusion of the sutures in the skull. The third cause is from prenatal or postnatal external constraint.[38]

The first of these is self-explanatory. If the brain is developing abnormally, or there is too much or too little fluid around the brain, it will put abnormal pressures on the skull. It is that internal pressure that gives the skull its irregular shape. An example of this is hydrocephalus, in which there is too much fluid around the brain, giving the head an enlarged appearance.

The second of these refers to the nature of the bones of the skull. Skull bones are not closed when a baby is born to allow him to pass through the birth canal, as well as to accommodate the growing brain as he matures. We call these open areas *fontanelles* or soft spots. As long as the soft spots are open, the head is molding and changing shape. We normally see these areas close around the first year to year and a half of life. Some close earlier, some later. When the soft spots close too early, it can result in an abnormally shaped head, because the brain is still trying to grow. This condition is called *craniosynostosis*.

The third cause of plagiocephaly refers to the external pressures on the skull either when the baby is in the womb or after he is born. In the womb, a baby can be crowded, because of a sibling sharing the same space, which is the case in multiple births. Alternatively, he could have been resting his head on his mother's pelvic bone, which can affect the shape of the head when he is born. Both are examples of prenatal constraint. During the birthing process, the baby's head typically molds into a cone shape in order for it to fit through the birth canal. This temporary molding typically resolves in the first week of life.[38]

Postnatal constraint is by far the most common cause of plagiocephaly. This is the pressure on the head from external sources like a crib mattress, the floor, or car seat. Positional plagiocephaly is the development of a flat spot on the back of the head or an abnormally shaped head due to outside pressure. Even if your baby was born through C-section with a nice, round head, plagiocephaly can still develop. There are different types of head deformation, but it has become commonplace to cluster all of these abnormalities in one group—plagiocephaly.

Positional plagiocephaly can develop when a baby spends a disproportionate amount of time on one part of the head while the soft spots are open. Researchers refer to this as a "forced sleeping position."[38] As you can imagine, it is referring to the exclusive habit of placing babies only on their backs. A flattening of the skull will develop on the side the baby lies upon most often. Furthermore, the brain grows in the path of least resistance; therefore it will grow away from the area of pressure.

Think of the brain as a tennis ball in a balloon filled with water. Since the walls of the balloon are soft, when you press on one side, the fluid pushes the ball to the other side. If the balloon becomes harder and you apply pressure, the ball and fluid have nowhere to go and get compressed. This is similar to the process of a baby's skull. In the beginning, it is not as hard and the soft spots are open, allowing the bones to move with displacement of fluid. As the baby matures and the soft spots close, the skull becomes harder, and there is no room for displacement.

There are three main types of positional plagiocephaly—brachycephaly, traditional plagiocephaly and scaphocephaly.

BRACHYCEPHALY

Brachycephaly is when the entire back of the skull flattens, with flaring of both ears. In my practice, I most often see brachycephaly when a baby has a tight trapezius muscle on both sides causing him to lie with his head directly in midline.

Head rotation is typically restricted on both sides in these cases.

Figure 5: Brachycephaly

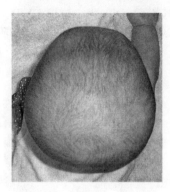

TRADITIONAL PLAGIOCEPHALY

The second type, traditional plagiocephaly, where the term "oblique head" comes from, is when the entire head is shifted on the diagonal, with the forehead protruding on one side and the opposite side of the back of the head flattened.[3] Accompanying this type of skull deformation are varying degrees of facial deformity, such as jaw flattening on one side with the eye on that side partially closed, flattening of the cheek bone, and ear flare.

Figure 6: Traditional Plagiocephaly

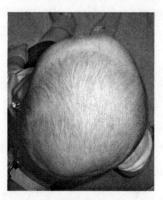

SCAPHOCEPHALY

The third type is scaphocephaly, where the head is oblong from front to back. Typically, treatment is not indicated for scaphocephaly, because the head is symmetrically rounded.

Figure 7: Scaphocephaly

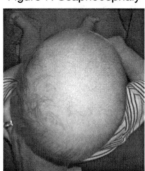

COMBINATION PLAGIOCEPHALY

A combination of brachycephaly and plagiocephaly can occur with both conditions appearing together. The head is both widened from side to side and shifted on a diagonal, with accompanying facial deformities. The flattening is typically worse on one side of the back of the head.

Figure 8: Combined Forms

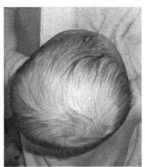

Positional plagiocephaly is worsened by gravitational forces, so lying on the back increases the likelihood of the head being deformed. The skull is developing at the fastest rate in the first year of life, an estimated 80 percent of lifetime growth.[3] It is therefore the most important time to ensure your baby's head is receiving equal forces on all sides.

There are other activities that contribute to positional plagiocephaly. Holding the baby on the same side to feed every time can be a causative factor. The increased use of car seats has also been associated with the rise in plagiocephaly cases. Babies who spend the majority of their time in a soft bouncer or swing to sleep, to eat, and to play are at high risk for head deformation because the soft surface does not require muscle strength to maintain a posture and allows the baby to sink into a favored resting position—typically with the head tilted to one side. In addition, the baby is receiving pressure only on the back of the head in all these apparatuses. Bones build strength by encountering a firm surface, and in keeping with the safe sleep environment, a firm surface is best. Car seats, bouncers, and swings tend to be soft and plush.

We tend to see torticollis and plagiocephaly together, because one can cause the other. Reports say this association is seen in 80-90 percent of cases.[36] For example, if a baby has spasmodic torticollis, he favors lying with his head turned to one side. Consistently lying on the same side of the head creates resistance on the back of the skull on that side, causing it to flatten. Once the skull is flattened, it is easier for the baby to continue to lie on that side, as rotating over the rounded part of the skull requires more muscle strength. Reciprocally, if a baby has developed plagiocephaly and continues to lie in the same way that caused it, the muscles will become shortened on that side of the neck creating the conditions for torticollis.

IMPLICATIONS ON DEVELOPMENT

The increased incidence of these two conditions is a major concern, because it has a strong influence on the child's development. The visual field can be affected if the eyes are not looking to both directions or are looking while tilted to one side. The field of vision influences development of the eye muscles and affects eye alignment. Visual problems can develop that could require intervention.

Orthodontic and TMJ (temporomandibular joint) problems can occur if concomitant facial deformities are left untreated. Developmental delay and muscle imbalances of the neck, back, and shoulder girdle can also be a result of torticollis, which could cause abnormal movement patterns. The effects may not even be seen until the child matures into adulthood and starts to experience orthopedic injury as a result.

In one study that tracked sixty-three families of children with persistent plagiocephaly, 39.7 percent required intervention by a physical therapist, occupational therapist, or speech therapist, or required special education assistance once they reached school age. This was compared to the 7.7 percent of siblings from the same family who required special services.[38]

Another report indicates there are long-term effects of plagiocephaly that present as language disorders, learning disabilities, and attention deficits when a child reaches school age due to compression of certain areas of the brain, if plagiocephaly is left untreated.[3]

Torticollis and plagiocephaly are also associated with sensory processing disorders. Also known as sensory integration disorders, these are conditions where the sensory system in the body is not processing or adapting to information that is coming in through the environment or within the body. This is any input that is perceived through the senses of sight, taste, smell, touch, balance, and coordination.

A sensory processing disorder for a baby with torticollis and plagiocephaly may present as over-sensitive or under-sensitive areas of the skin on the head and face. It may present as either poor vision or, alternatively, the ability to give meaning to what is seen.

If the baby is in one position most of the time, the inner ear—or vestibular—sense may not get a chance to adapt to movement of the head. The different positions of development help mature this sense of balance as the body works against gravity. Babies who have an underdeveloped vestibular or balance sense may be overly clumsy or avoid activities with a lot of movement.

PREVENTION AND INTERVENTION

Now that you know what causes torticollis and plagiocephaly and the effects it can have on a child, how do you prevent these conditions from occurring? As positional torticollis and plagiocephaly are much more prevalent today due to the Back to Sleep campaign, it is important to pay attention to and address which position the baby is in on a regular basis, ensuring that no one position takes precedence!

The best way to do this is to place your baby on a firm surface such as a crib, play yard, bassinet, or on a thin blanket or sheet on the floor during sleep and play to allow the tensile strength of the bones to develop. A firm surface will also reduce the risk of suffocation and/or SIDS. Second, rotate his position throughout the day, so he is lying on a different part of his head. The different positions I am talking about are . . .

- Side-lying on the right,
- Side-lying on the left,
- Lying on the back, and
- Lying on the stomach.

This rotation of your baby's position not only helps ensure a well-rounded head, but it also ensures well-balanced muscle development. If you are uncomfortable with placing your baby on his side or stomach, only do so during the day under your supervision. And, when your baby is on his back, make sure to turn his head to each side while he sleeps to deter a favored sleeping position.

If you are bottle-feeding your baby, remember to alternate the side you hold him on just as you would when breastfeeding, to encourage head rotation to each side. This will both help to develop his eyes as he looks at you and encourage muscle balance of his neck.

Parents have told me that the doctor assured them the head deformation will go away on its own over time. This cannot be further from the truth. Plagiocephaly will not resolve by itself if nothing changes about the way the infant is cared for. If he continues to lie in the favored position, the plagiocephaly—and torticollis—will get worse. You cannot expect a positive outcome unless you change the pattern of forces on the baby's head by positioning him in different ways. You also cannot expect a baby to develop balanced muscle strength unless the muscles are given an opportunity to move against gravity in different positions.

In the event your baby does develop torticollis or plagiocephaly or both, your doctor may refer you to a physical therapist for an evaluation. During the evaluation, the PT will assess the shape of your baby's head and determine the amount of range of motion he has in his neck. After assessment, the PT will give you an exercise program for stretching the neck muscles and a positioning program to round out the shape of your baby's head.

Early identification and treatment of the baby's condition is the first key to a successful outcome; the second is the parents' full compliance with and participation in the stretching and positioning programs designed to address the condition. Your therapist will know if you are compliant with the stretching and positioning programs. Trust me, I know!

The good news is that 95 percent of torticollis cases resolve within one year with a stretching program.[36] I encourage all my parents to continue monitoring their baby's neck motion throughout the first year, because each time a growth spurt occurs, it is possible for the muscles to get a bit tight again. This usually resolves by one year old, because the baby is moving about on his own and doing all the stretching that needs to be done in the process.

Plagiocephaly usually resolves by the first six months to one year with a positioning program. Again, the earlier the baby is treated for head deformity, the faster and more successful is the rounding of the skull. Positioning techniques have reduced the flattening and shifting of the skull to *mild* or *normal* in

100 percent of my patients. Mild is when there is less than a centimeter difference from the left side of the skull to the right side, measured on a diagonal. Normal is when there is negligible or no difference from one side to the other on measurement.

Proper positioning therapy has also reduced the facial deformity and ear asymmetry to mild or normal in 100 percent of my patients. This means the forehead protrusion resolves and the ears appear level and/or near equal in flare. I speak from experience when I tell you that positioning programs do work if the parents follow through with them.

Before and After

Below are pictures of one of my patients who displayed the typical results of a parent who actively participated in the positioning program. Initially, he had moderate flattening of the back of the right side of his head, with forehead protrusion on the right. After just a month of positioning, the flattening reduced to mild and the forehead protrusion resolved.

Figure 9: Before

Figure 10: After

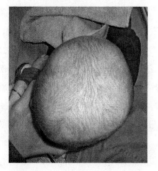
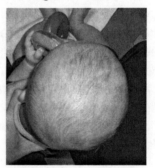

Orthotics Options

For babies who do not have this success with positioning, there is the option of a cranial remolding helmet or headband. You may or may not have seen a baby with one of these orthoses, but it looks just like it sounds—a helmet! It works by maintaining the high points or rounded areas of the skull, with the theory that the brain will grow in the path of least resistance, thus rounding out flattened areas. Optimally, the helmet is fit before the baby is nine months old and is worn anywhere from two to nine months, depending on the severity of the head deformity. The baby wears the helmet for twenty-three hours a day, and you must return to an orthotist or other cranial remolding specialist periodically for adjustments and to monitor progress.[39]

There are several different orthotic companies that make cranial remodeling helmets or headbands. Likely, the orthotist you visit will have a preference for a particular company and product. It is important for you to know that treatment with head-remolding orthotics can cost up to $3,000. Some insurance companies cover this cost, but others consider plagiocephaly a cosmetic issue and will not cover it. I encourage you to check with your insurance company before deciding on any treatment program and determine any out-of-pocket costs you may incur.

The process varies slightly between clinics, but usually a cast or digital picture will be taken of the skull to custom-fit the helmet for your child. The casting process involves applying strips of plaster to the baby's head, waiting a few moments while it dries, and then removing it. This gives the orthotist a three-dimensional plaster impression of your child's head. A newer approach is a computer scan, which involves placing the infant inside the scanner where lasers and cameras create a digital picture of the baby's head. Both of these procedures are noninvasive and should not cause any discomfort to your child.

Another orthotic option is the tubular orthosis for torticollis or TOT collar. This cervical or neck orthotic is used when a child's head tilt does not resolve with stretching and exercise. It consists of two rubber tubes with plastic stays that are adjusted to support the neck on the affected side in the neutral position. This treatment approach is only appropriate for children four months and older, and unlike the helmet, the TOT collar is only worn while the child is awake. It works by providing a noxious stimulus to one side of the neck, which causes the baby to move away from that side to a more upright position.[40]

The drawback of the TOT collar is its tendency to lose its position if the child is moving around. The plastic stays are designed to give a stimulus in one spot, but being a collar, it can easily migrate around the neck, rendering it ineffective in the area that needs stimulating.

Other Treatment Options

On rare occasions, surgical intervention is used to treat torticollis. This is only indicated when the child is over one year old and all conservative methods have not worked, particularly if there is a lack of fifteen degrees of rotation of the neck after six months of manual stretching. Children who seek treatment at older ages are more likely to require surgery to release the tightened SCM muscle.

Surgery is also an option for head deformity when all conservative treatment methods have failed or produced less-than-desired results.[36] This is more often the case with *craniosynostosis,* in which the sutures or soft spots of the skull close prematurely, and abnormalities like hydrocephalus, in which there is excess fluid around the brain.

Botox (Botulinum toxin) injections have also been used on rare occasions to relax the involved muscles for stretching and to allow strengthening of the weak, over-stretched muscles on the opposite side.

Torticollis and Plagiocephaly are treatable diagnoses, but the best treatment is prevention. It is possible to prevent these two conditions and still reduce the risk of SIDS. Following the safety guidelines regarding sleep environment along with the practice of alternating the position of your baby will help ensure a favorable outcome. You, the caregivers, are the key to success in reducing the rising number of infants who are diagnosed with torticollis and plagiocephaly each day.

8

DEVELOPMENTAL DELAY

Developmental delay has many causes. It would be incorrect to assume the lack of tummy time is the only reason for a baby to be behind in meeting motor milestones. The underlying conditions for delay are numerous and not within the scope of this book. We will therefore only discuss developmental delay as related to the Back to Sleep program.

Any delay in development will be diagnosed by a pediatrician following certain guidelines. By definition, developmental delay is when a child does not meet one or more milestones by the accepted "normal" range of time. For instance, the normal range for walking is between nine and fifteen months of age. If a twenty-month-old child is not walking, this is considered a developmental delay.[41] Oftentimes, other issues are going on with the child as well. There may be a pattern of meeting all milestones "a little late." But remember, prematurity and adjusted age will also determine when your child should meet milestones.

Since the start of the Back to Sleep program, there has been a steady increase in the number of children that are developmentally delayed. This delay can be mild to severe, meaning that some children may be just a bit behind their peers or several months behind their peers who are the same age. Below is a chart that tracks the rise of this diagnosis during the same years as the Back to Sleep program.

Figure 11: Developmental Delay Chart[43]

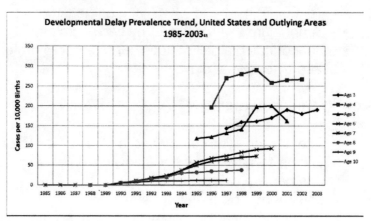

It would be correct to assume that this increase in the number of children who are developmentally delayed is due to babies spending the majority of time on their backs and not developing muscle strength in all areas of the body. You are now well aware that the best way to develop this balance is by placing your baby in different lying positions.

The following are some warning signs of developmental delay that health professionals use as a screening tool for infants. Please, remember that every child develops at her own pace—if she is doing (or not doing) some of the things on this list, it does not necessarily mean there is a delay. Health professionals look for a pattern in these areas to determine a potential problem. Here are some things to look for if you are concerned about your child:

GROSS MOTOR WARNING SIGNS

- Has stiff arms and/or legs that are difficult to move
- Has floppy arms or legs, a limp body when picked up and moved
- Uses one side of the body more than the other/does not use one arm or leg

- Clumsy, falls more frequently than other children of the same age
- Cannot lift her head when lying on her stomach
- Cannot jump with two feet by two years old
- Cannot catch a ball or does not attempt to protect her face by one year old

VISION WARNING SIGNS

- One or both eyes seem abnormal in size or color
- Seems to have difficulty following objects or people with her eyes after infancy
- Squints or rubs eyes frequently
- Turns, tilts head in a strained or abnormal position when looking at an object or holds object very close to the face
- Appears to have difficulty finding a small object dropped on the ground after one year old
- Has difficulty focusing on an object or making eye contact
- Closes one eye when trying to look at an object that is far away
- Eyes appear to be crossed or turned or one eye lags behind the other

HEARING WARNING SIGNS

- Talks very loudly or very softly
- Difficulty hearing name when called from a distance/ does not respond
- Turns her body so that the same ear is always toward the sound
- Has a difficult time understanding what is said or following verbal instructions
- Is not bothered by loud noises that bother other children
- Is delayed in speech that is age appropriate—is more difficult to understand than other children her age

FINE-MOTOR WARNING SIGNS

- Unable to pick up small objects with first finger and thumb by one year old
- Holds pencil/crayon with an awkward grip by six years old
- Does not display a hand dominance by preschool
- Leans on forearms while coloring or eating or props self up with arms
- Cannot manipulate scissors by school age
- Difficulty getting dressed—difficulty with buckles, snaps, Velcro, zippers, tying shoes by six years old.[41]

VESTIBULAR/BALANCE WARNING SIGNS

- Afraid of swings, elevators, escalators, slides—anything that moves
- Gets motion sickness easily
- Holds head and neck in a stiff position
- Cautious with movement OR
- Craves constant motion—spinning, being upside down, fidgeting, inability to sit still

Developmental delay is screened by your pediatrician in a few different ways. One that you may be familiar with is a written questionnaire given to you to answer about your child when you go in for a well-child visit. You answer yes/no questions about the skills your child demonstrates an ability to do. Your child's doctor reviews your responses and determines if your baby is developing on target. The pediatrician may also have your child perform a few skills during the check-up like standing on one foot and running across the room, if age appropriate. If the doctor determines that your child may be delayed, a referral will be made to another professional who specializes in that area of concern. For example, if a gross motor delay is suspected, a referral may be made to a physical therapist. If a vision issue is identified, a referral may be made to an optometrist or ophthalmologist. And of course, if a speech delay is detected, a referral may be made to a speech/language pathologist (also called a speech therapist). If you have specific concerns about your child, do not hesitate to discuss them with your pediatrician. This will help the process along and can only benefit your child.

As a PT, I see many developmentally delayed children. Of these, some are patients who I previously treated for torticollis and plagiocephaly. There appears to be a direct correlation between how active the parents were with the positioning and stretching programs and whether they returned to therapy with concerns of delay. The vast majority of patients I see with torticollis and plagiocephaly, whose parents engage in routinely stretching and positioning them, come back at the one-month checkup with vast improvements in range of motion and reduced plagiocephaly, as well as progression with their developmental milestones.

Once allowed to spend time on her stomach, a baby builds strength quickly and discovers she can do many things. Parents report rolling that did not occur before, pivoting on the stomach, attempting to sit up, among other things. The older a child is when she is initially brought into PT for a torticollis or plagiocephaly evaluation, the more likely one or more of the milestones have not been met. Conversely, the earlier I see a baby for these two conditions, the less likely she will experience any delay in milestone acquisition.

Avoiding the Skipped Milestone

I am often asked about a baby skipping a milestone. Most commonly, people say that their baby never crawled but went straight to walking. This is something I caution against. Each skill builds on the next one and serves its own purpose. Rolling builds strength in the muscles on the sides of the trunk as well as muscles in the neck. If a baby skips rolling, a weakness could develop in the trunk and neck muscles. If a baby skips crawling, she is missing out on the strengthening of shoulder girdle and hips that occurs from being on all fours. Crawling is essential for establishing the right brain-left brain connection that will later be used for reading and writing, as well as cross-body skills.

Crawling on all fours also develops the arches of the hands necessary for handwriting and many other manual skills later on. Many advocates state that *crawling is the most important developmental milestone,* because it coordinates the arms and legs with movement of the head. The result is a well-coordinated child who moves her arms, legs, and head independently.[43]

From a clinical standpoint, I love crawling! I tell the parents of every child I see to encourage crawling *no matter what their age*. The benefits of crawling are huge! So when a parent tells me that their child was an early walker and never crawled, I cringe a little. Of all the skills to skip, please, don't let your children skip crawling. What I am saying is please, don't encourage or *practice* walking with your child before she has crawled for at least two months or more. In a perfect world, a child wouldn't skip any skill, because each is a building block for the next. A child will find any way to accomplish her movement goal, even if it means moving in an unusual way, which could put her at risk for developing muscle imbalances and weaknesses.

Something else to consider is that a baby may have a weakness that hinders her from successfully accomplishing the milestone, so she skips it all together. She will use compensatory movements to accomplish her movement goals, thus hiding the muscle imbalance. Whether it is a muscle or group of muscles that are not working properly or a joint that does not have full range of motion, the baby will work around it. For you, this may just be her "cute way of doing that," but in the long term, she is building on improper movements, which could make your child prone to injury in the future or unsuccessful in accomplishing future milestones.

EARLY INTERVENTION AND THE IEP

If you suspect that your child is developmentally delayed either as a result of torticollis and plagiocephaly or for some other reason, there are many resources out there to help you. The first step is to talk to your child's doctor about your concerns. The doctor will examine your child and refer you to a facility or agency. Early intervention is a service that is provided by public agencies or private organizations for children under three years old. Each state has its own regulations and programs for early intervention. Some of the resources provided are physical therapy, occupational therapy, speech therapy, psychological services, nutrition services, and nursing services just to name a few. If a child qualifies for these services, an individualized education program (IEP) will be written.

An IEP is a federally mandated written report that outlines a child's disabilities, current level of function, current academic performance, and specific needs. Included in this report are the annual goals and objectives for that child. After an IEP is established, a team decides which services the child requires.[41] The treatments usually involve the relevant professional coming to your home for therapy visits. For more information, about early intervention and IEPs, check with your doctor about the services available in your area.

Another option might be a referral to a hospital or private facility for therapy services. This referral typically comes from a pediatrician. In a hospital or private facility, a team of people are often available to evaluate your child. Typically, a physical therapist, occupational therapist, speech therapist, and sometimes a psychologist are on staff at these facilities. Which professionals you see will depend on your child's needs. Each profession brings its own evaluation process to the table to identify key goals for its area of expertise. For example, a physical therapist will evaluate physical limitations and establish treatment goals based on the individual child's needs and the goals of the parents.

If your child is old enough, he may be referred to a school-based setting to receive physical therapy, occupational therapy, and/or speech therapy. In conjunction with early intervention, children qualify for school therapy at age three in the United States. These programs were developed as a result of the Individuals with Disabilities Act (IDEA) originating in 1975. This federal law governs how state and public agencies provide special services, such as early intervention and special education to children with disabilities. Children from birth to age twenty-one qualify for these services. There have been several revisions since the original act with the most recent revisions done in 2004. This specified that every child with a disability must be provided with free public education to prepare them for the future. IDEA is considered a civil right, but each state is not required to participate and has its own rules and regulations.[44] To learn more about your own state's IDEA regulations, contact your local school board.

Developmental delay as related to the Back to Sleep program and sleep positioning is treatable, but again, the best treatment is prevention. This is best achieved by giving your baby opportunity to move and develop unhindered. You, the caregivers, can help reduce the number of children who are diagnosed each day with developmental delay by starting with your own child in this manner.

9

CAR SEATS AND CONFINEMENT

With the dawn of the safety age, car seats have arrived on the scene with much exuberance. If you walk around the mall or any other highly populated area, you will see numerous strollers with car seats clipped on the top or parents hauling their babies around in the car seat itself. Often, babies are not even taken out to be fed or to have their diapers changed. The bottle is just inserted in its proper place and the baby eats, sleeps, and observes the world from this stationary capsule. Yes, they are very convenient to parents, because their babies are contained. They have the ease of being clipped into a base in the car. They have the convenience of being clipped into a stroller, and they have the expediency of being carried around as a portable baby transporter. Unfortunately, car seats are leading to a whole slew of problems for developing babies.

Even though the car seat has been moved several times a day, the baby has not. While strapped into the car seat, your baby is confined on his back without having to use one muscle to move around, except perhaps moving his arms to bat at the numerous toys attached to the handle. Not only is the baby not using muscles to explore his world, he is also getting a very limited view of the environment; hence, his eyes have few opportunities to develop. Lying on his back, confined in a car seat, a baby is not allowed much change in his head position, therefore limiting the stimulation to the vestibular or balance system. And last, but certainly not least, because the baby is not being held by a warm person, he is missing out on all of the benefits of touching another human being.

Along with the increased use of car seats is the dramatic decrease in floor time for infants. This would be free playtime on the floor, crib, or play yard, with just a sheet or thin blanket on which the baby is allowed to move freely in her environment. Even newborn babies move a lot if placed on the floor. Remember that all of this movement is giving the baby messages about the world around her, teaching her how to use her muscles, her head, and her eyes to experience all the different sensations.

The current trend is to always have the baby contained in some sort of contraption. These include, but are not limited to swings, bouncers, Exersaucers, tummy mats, and the whole array of other devices manufacturers are insisting are essential for good development. What do all of these items have in common? They confine the baby so she doesn't have to use her muscles to do anything. She is passively entertained by the sparkling, flashing toy in front of her, forcing her to be an observer instead of actively participating in the activity. Parents may be fooled into believing that the tummy mats are helping their children develop on their stomachs, but again, the baby is propped up by the chest cushion and looking down at the mat instead of using her shoulder muscles to prop on her arms and her neck and back muscles to lift her head to see what is around her.

Not only do these items confine babies and prevent muscle use, they also are typically soft. Soft material, especially on the stomach, exponentially increases the risk for SIDS, as we have seen. Confinement also prevents reflexes from becoming integrated, preventing babies from developing normally. Consistent pressure from a car seat, bouncer, or swing also contributes to plagiocephaly, as the favored position in these apparatuses contributes to torticollis. If a baby is not using her muscles, she will likely not meet developmental milestones on time.

Most parents believe that a baby should just progress through development without any help and often express their confusion when they come to physical therapy with their baby. Here is the explanation: a baby will typically develop on his own through the use of reflexes and muscle strength against gravity, if he is allowed free play on the floor, unrestricted. If he is confined through the phases that these reflexes are engaged to prompt movement and voluntary muscle use, the window of opportunity is missed and the movements may have to be taught, the reflexes addressed. Obviously, if the baby has special needs, this may not be the case. However, we are talking here about a typical baby with no underlying problems.

We can continue to add to the list of problems that confinement causes by including sensory integration problems. The senses—touch, taste, hearing, vision, balance—develop by movement, exploration, and position change. If a baby is in the same position most of the time, these senses may not develop or may send an incorrect message to the brain because of what is occurring too often or too seldom. A sensory integration issue can be created. If a baby is limited in feeling sensations like being held, feeling the pull of gravity on her joints, balancing to keep her head upright, or feeling the different textures of the floor as she moves about, her sensory system can be compromised. If a baby is consistently restricted from putting things in her mouth, she could develop an oral integration issue. Putting things in their mouths is how babies learn about them. They feel the texture, the shape, the temperature, and the taste of objects with their mouths, and explore them with their eyes and hands. If a baby is not often held, the sensation of being hugged or being touched could be so unfamiliar that it is uncomfortable. You can see how if a baby is confined, she is missing out on this exploration that is essential to normal development.

A parent brought her adopted son to see me for developmental delay and sensory processing disorder. She told me a horror story of how he was tied to his crib in the orphanage to prevent him from moving around. This child also had untreated plagiocephaly, but at age four, there was nothing short of surgery to correct it. He was now experiencing the effects of being confined and required intervention. The lack of movement and stimulation adopted children have sometimes experienced often leads to developmental delay, sensory processing disorder, and deformed head shape, among other issues. When you compare this to the confinement of car seats, bouncers, swings, etc., the results are sadly similar. Though the reasons for the confinement are different, both sets of children will ultimately suffer the consequences of confinement.

Not only is the constant use of a car seat bad for the baby, it can also be bad for the parent. Many parents complain to me about horrible neck, back, and shoulder pain from lugging around a car seat with a baby in it all the time. The combined weight of a fifteen-pound baby and a car seat is too much weight to carry on one side of your body. It's enough of a workout to make anyone sore.

I recommend using car seats only in the car! Consider a sling that wraps over your shoulder or a front/backpack carrier as better methods for transporting your baby. These are fabulous because the baby is not only close to you for comfort, but also upright! He will have to use his muscles against gravity and will get to work on balance. When you lean forward or sideways, he is receiving input to the vestibular/balance sense. If he is forward facing, he can see what is happening around him. His arms and legs are free to explore. And best of all, you are holding him. A great deal of research confirms the benefit of physical touch on the emotional security an infant. By being next to you, he gets that sense of emotional security and nurturing. Furthermore, carriers and slings free your arms without putting excessive strain on your back and neck.

I even recommend putting your baby in a stroller *without the car seat attached*. The manufacturers make every kind of stroller these days. If your infant doesn't have the strength or control to sit fully upright, recline her so she is supported. Many stroller backs become a bassinet when completely reclined. You can put your baby on her back or side, or even her stomach, with your watchful eye monitoring her. You can't do that in a car seat.

It is not to say that babies can never spend any time in bouncers, car seats, swings, or the like; they just shouldn't spend most of their time there. The majority of your baby's time should be spent on a firm surface on a thin blanket or sheet, in different positions (stomach, each side, and back), or being held. Occasional use of a swing, car seat, bouncer, or other device will not be detrimental. The key thing to think about is position variety.

In summary, please, only put your baby in the car seat when in the car and use swings, bouncers, and so on sparingly. It will not only be better for your baby, but better for you as well. The period of development in the first year is so brief. Before you know it, your baby will be walking everywhere you go.

10

CONCLUSION

In this era of convenience and being passive participants to entertainment, it is essential that we are diligently conscious of the development of our children. It is of paramount importance to continue the "old fashioned" ways of allowing our children unstructured, free playtime on the floor during the vital first year of life. It is during this first year that infants learn so many skills that will benefit them for the rest of their lives. In the scope of one year, a baby goes from being born helpless and completely dependent on others for his care to controlling his head, his body, his fingers, and toes, and then is either walking or close to walking. That is a huge step from beginning to end!

Knowledge is power, and with the information presented on SIDS and the Back to Sleep program, I hope you are now ready to abate your fears about the position you place your baby in. Current technology exists to screen your baby for potential problem areas. If you are still concerned, I encourage you to seek professional advice for your peace of mind and for your baby's well being.

Movement is essential not only for development, but also to help prevent things like torticollis, plagiocephaly, developmental delay, sensory processing disorder, and related conditions. Confinement is the exact opposite of movement. And although convenient, the use of car seats, bouncers, swings, and related baby containers oppose movement.

Keeping with the "old fashioned" way of learning, I encourage you to seek out toys that require the child to be active in playing with them, instead of the other way around where the child is a passive participant to flashing lights, moving pictures, sounds, and all manner of machine activity. I often take the batteries out of toys in my clinic to teach children the value of being satisfied with the simple cause and effect of a toy without all the bells and whistles. The more engaged a child is in playing, the more developed his brain will become. Remember that children lose their motivation to progress if they are passive participants in the learning process, because their brains are not stimulated into movement. Watching TV, playing video games and other hand-held gaming systems only encourage a constant flash of movement in a child's eyes, but do not require the child to move. The likelihood of developing to the highest potential physically and mentally all begins in that first year and is directly linked to how much opportunity for movement is provided, how many positions the baby explores, and whether the reflexes are allowed to play the role for which they are intended. Help your baby reach the highest level of achievement. You are the key to success.

References

1. Cech D., S. Martin. *Functional Movement Development Across the Life Span*. Philadelphia, PA: W.B. Saunders Company, 1995.
2. Blomberg, Harald and Moira Dempsey. *Rhythmic Movement Training*. (2006) US Edition Revised March 2008. www.rhythmicmovement.com.
3. Folio, Rhonda M., and Rebecca R. Fewell. *Peabody Developmental Motor Scales,* second edition, Austin, TX: PRO-ED, (1983) 2000.
4. Julie C. *Plagiocephaly and Torticollis: Causes and Effects on Alignment and Development*. December 2, 2005. http://www.epinions.com/content_4587102340.
5. Bundonis, Joanne. "Benefits of Early Mobility with Emphasis on Gait Training", *Rifton Equipment,* 2009, www.rifton.com/adaptive-mobility-blog
6. Anderson, Kenneth. *Mosby's Medical, Nursing and Allied Health Dictionary*, fourth edition. St. Louis, MO: Mosby-Year Book, Inc., 1994.
7. Kochanek, Kenneth D. et al. "Deaths: Preliminary Data for 2009." *National Vital Statistics Reports* Volume 59, Number 4. March 16, 2011.
8. NIH/NICHD (General Outreach). "Safe Sleep for Your Baby: Ten Ways to Reduce the Risk of Sudden Infant Death Syndrome (SIDS)." NIH Pub. No. 05-7040 (October 2005) Updated August 13, 2009. http://www.nichd.nih.gov/publications/pubs/safe_sleep_gen.cfm.

9. Kattwinkel, John et al. American Academy of Pediatrics Policy Statement. "The Changing Concept of Sudden Infant Death Syndrome: Diagnostic Coding Shifts, Controversies Regarding the Sleeping Environment, and New Variables to Consider in Reducing Risk." *Pediatrics* November. 2005. 116 (5): 1245-1255.
10. Doheny, Kathleen. "Low Serotonin Levels May Be Key to SIDS." *Health and Baby,* February 2, 2010.
11. Ghatak, Ashim, MD, et al. "Serotonin: Ubiquitous Neuromodulator in the Failing Heart." *Asian Cardiovascular and Thoracic Annals,* 1998; 6: 11-16.
12. "Bundle of His." Wikipedia, the free encyclopedia; www.wikipedia.org.
13. Bharati, Krongrad E., M. Lev. "Study of the Conduction System in Population of Patients with Sudden Infant Death Syndrome." *Pediatric Cardiology.* Springer-Verlag, 1985.
14. Lie, J. T., H. S. Rosenberg, and E. E. Erickson. "Histopathology of Conduction System in the Sudden Infant Death Syndrome." *Circulation.* 53: 3-8. American Heart Association, 1976.
15. Ewer, A. K. "Pulse Oximetry as a Screening Test for Congenital Heart Disease in Newborn Babies." NIHR Health Technology Assessment Programme. December 23, 2008. http://www.hta.ac.uk/1624.
16. Jancin, B. "Screening for Long QT Syndrome May Cut SIDS." *Pediatric News,* July, 2005.
17. Mayo Foundation for Medical Education and Research. "Heart Disease: Long QT Syndrome." www.MayoClinic.com/health/long-qt-syndrome/DS00434.
18. U.S. Department of Health and Human Services, National Institutes of Health. "What Causes Long QT Syndrome?" *National Heart Lung and Blood Institute Diseases and Conditions Index.* www.nhlbi.nih.gov/health/dci/Diseases/qt/qt_causes.html.
19. Silverman, Ed. *Antidepressants + Pregnancy= Higher Risks: Study.* November 5, 2009; www.pharmalot.

com/2009/11/antidepressants-pregnancy-higher-risks-study/.

20. Mayo Foundation for Medical Education and Research. "Antidepressants: Safe During Pregnancy?" *Pregnancy Week by Week,* December 17, 2009, 1998-2011.

21. Hunter's Hope Foundation. *Why is Universal Newborn Screening Important for All Babies?* Hunter's Hope Foundation brochure, 2008. www.huntershope.org.

22. Woo, Joseph. *Obstetric Ultrasound: A Comprehensive Guide.* www.ob-ultrasound.net.

23. US Department of Health and Human Resources. *Congenital Heart Defects.* NIH brochure. Revised August 2009.

24. About Kids Health News. *Should We Screen Every Child at Birth for a Rare Heart Condition?* www.aboutkidshealth.com/news.

25. Saving Babies through Screening Foundation, Inc. "Screening Information: How Do I Get Additional Screening for My Child?" Updated September 9, 2008. Save Babies Through Screening Foundation brochure, 2008. www.savebabies.org.

26. University of London, School of Hygiene and Tropical Medicine. "Simple Interventions Could Dramatically Reduce Rates of Cot Death in Europe." January 16, 2004. www.lshtm.ac.uk/news/2004/sidsreport.html.

27. NIH/NICHD. "Bed Sharing with Siblings, Soft Bedding, Increase SIDS Risk and Frequently Asked Questions about Bed Sharing." NIH/NICHD News Release, May 5, 2003. Updated September 16, 2008. www.nichd.nih.gov/news/releases/sidsRisk.cfm.

28. Carroll, J. *SIDS, Suffocation, Asphyxia, and Sleeping Position.* www.sids-network.org/experts/carroll2.htm.

29. Hargrove, T., L. Bowman. *Many Babies Die from Suffocation, not SIDS, Study Shows.* Scripps Howard News Service, December 16, 2007.

30. Shapiro-Mendoza, et al. "US Infant Mortality Trends Attributable to Accidental Suffocation and Strangulation

in Bed from 1984 through 2004: Are Rates Increasing?" *Pediatrics* 123 (2): 533-539, February 2009.

31. U.S. Central Intelligence Agency. "Country Comparison: Infant Mortality Rate" *The World Factbook* 2010. www.cia.gov.

32. MacDorman, Marian F., T. J. Mathews. *Recent Trends in Infant Mortality in the United State,s* NCHS Data Brief Number 9, October 2008.

33. MacDorman, Marian F., and T. J. Mathews. "Recent Trends in Infant Mortality in the United States." *NCHS Data Brief.* CDC No. 9, October 2008.

34. MedicineNet.com. "Infant Mortality" *Healthy Kids and Pediatrics* www.medicinenet.com

35. Morrow, Angela. "Leading Causes of Infant Death—Infant Mortality in the United States." July 27, 2009, www.about.com.

36. Szabo, Liz. "Study: Babies' Low Serotonin Levels Cause SIDS." *USA Today*, February 2, 2010.

37. Freed, S. S., C. Coulter-O'Berry. "Identification and Treatment of Congenital Muscular Torticollis in Infants." *American Academy of Orthotists and Prosthetists Journal of Prosthetics & Orthotics,* 2004; 16 (4S): 18-23.

38. Williams, C. R. P., et al. "Torticollis Secondary to Ocular Pathology." South Hampton University Hospital, England. *Bone Joint Surgery BR,* 1996; 78-B (620):4

39. Miller, R., S. K. Clarren. "Long-Term Developmental Outcomes in Patients with Deformational Plagiocephaly." *Pediatrics* 105 (2) 26. February 2000.

40. Midwest Orthotics & Technology Center. *Cranial Remolding* brochure 2001.

41. *The TOT Collar (Tubular Orthosis for Torticollis),* 2009. www.AliMed.com.

42. CASRC. "What Is Developmental Delay and What Services Are Available If I Think My Child Might Be Delayed?" *How Kids Develop.* 2008. CASRC. www.howkidsdevelop.com/developdevdelay.html.

43. Thoughtful House Center for Children. "Developmental Delay—Statistics, Incidence, Prevalence, Rates." Austin,

Texas: *Thoughtful House Center for Children.* 2010. www.thoughtfulhouse.org/tech-labs/disabilities/rates.

44. Myomancy. "How Important is Crawling as a Developmental Milestone?" *Myomancy ADHD, Dyslexia and Autism.* www.myomancy.com/2006/08.

45. US Department of Education. *Building the Legacy: IDEA 2004.* www.idea.ed.gov.

Additional Resources

Ackerman, M.J., et. al. "Postmortem Molecular Analysis of SCN5A Defects in Sudden Infant Death Syndrome." *JAMA* 2001; 286:2264-2269.

Baby Center Medical Advisory Board. *Milestone Chart 1 to 6 months and Milestone Chart 7 to 12 months.* Updated September 2006. Baby Center, LLC. 1997-2009. www.babycenter.com.

Bryant, Liz. "Serotonin levels linked to SIDS." February 4, 2010. FourStatesHomePage.com.

Keep Kids Healthy, LLC. "Developmental Delays," 1999-2009. www.keepkidshealthy.com.

Linwood, A. S. "Developmental Delay." *Children's Health Encyclopedia: Developmental Delay* 2009. www.Answers.com.

Miller, M.D., J. C., Porter, M. J. Ackerman. "Diagnostic Accuracy of Screening Electrocardiograms in Long QT Syndrome I." *Pediatrics* 108 (1): 8-12, July 2001.

Moon, Rachel Y., et al. "Sudden Infant Death Syndrome in Child Care Settings." *Pediatrics* 106 (2): 295-300, August 2000.

Sudden Unexplained Death in Childhood (SUDC) Program website 2007-2010. www.sudc.org.

Winchester, Sara. "Retained Primitive Reflexes." Total Chiropractic. www.totalchiro.com.

CPSIA information can be obtained at www.ICGtesting.com
Printed in the USA
LVOW131259110412

277164LV00001B/4/P